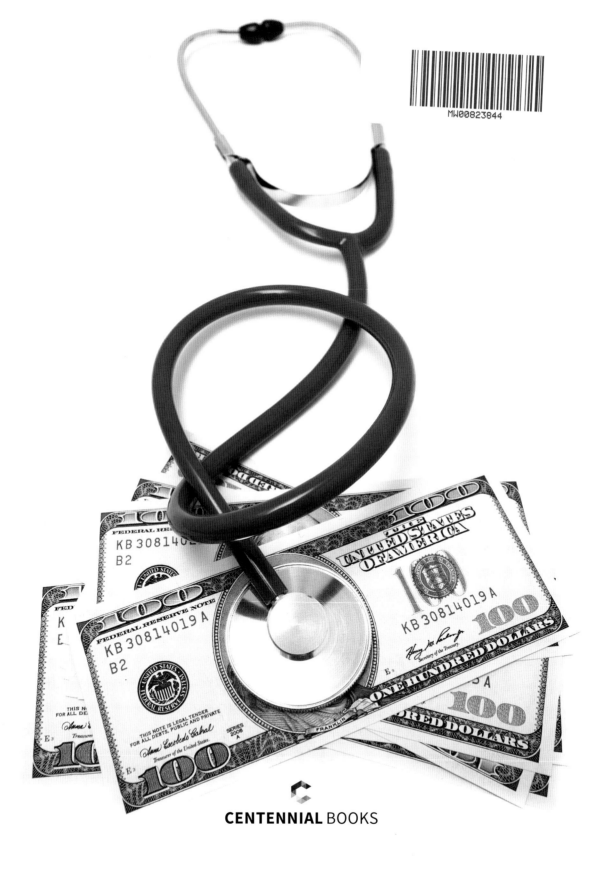

CENTENNIAL BOOKS

Take the Pain Out of

Medicare

Contents

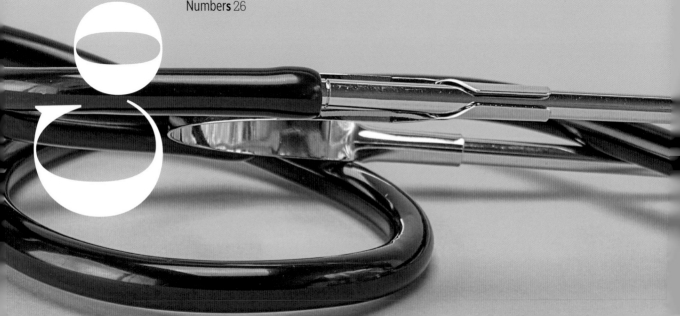

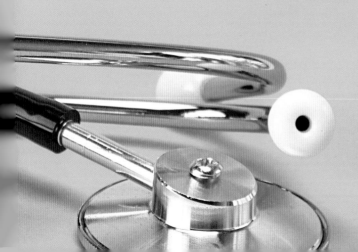

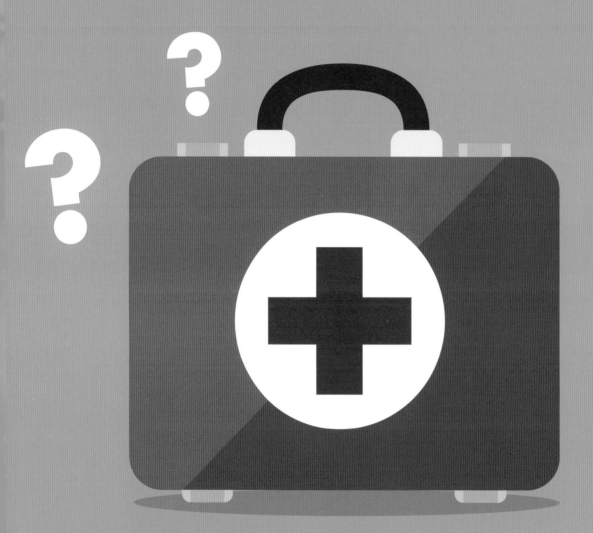

What Is Medicare?

An overview of the U.S. government's
health-insurance program for seniors

MEDICARE: AN OVERVIEW This government program has a lot to offer—especially if you understand how it works

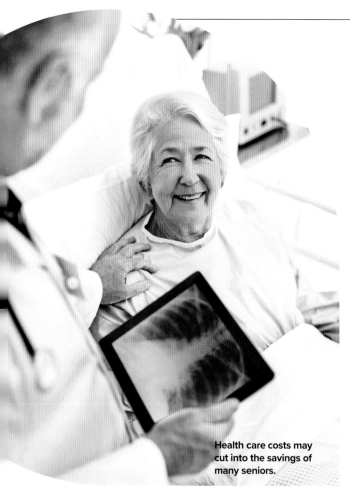

Health care costs may cut into the savings of many seniors.

As we age, our health care costs increase. We go to the doctor more often, require more prescription medications and sometimes need in-home care. However, for many of us, aging also means living on a fixed income—relying on Social Security and savings to cover our living expenses. Medicare was created to help seniors pay for increasingly expensive health care costs without going broke. It's an important government program that today provides health insurance for more than 60 million people.

If you're confused about how Medicare works, you're not alone. Many people planning for retirement struggle to understand all of the program's ins and outs. It doesn't cover everything, and as with all health insurance, there's plenty of fine print.

The Basics

At its core, Medicare is a basic health insurance program provided by the federal government. Most Medicare recipients are seniors—people 65

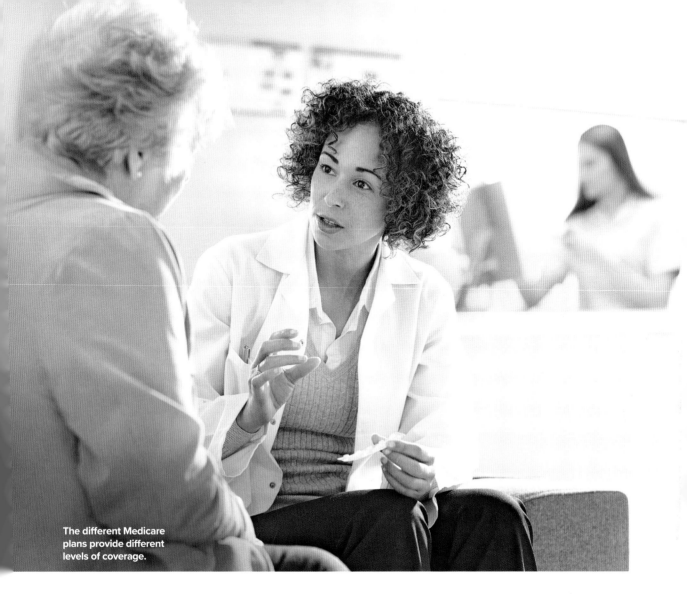

The different Medicare plans provide different levels of coverage.

or older. However, people with certain disabilities or illnesses can also qualify regardless of age. Because Medicare is administered by the federal government, there are no state-by-state eligibility requirements, although some benefits may vary depending on where you live.

For most people, Medicare will cut the costs of health care significantly. However, what's known as "Original Medicare" doesn't cover everything, and you'll still have out-of-pocket costs. These costs can be substantial if you don't choose a plan wisely, or if you fail to anticipate what your health care needs might be in the future, so it's essential to research your options.

Learn Your ABCs (and Ds)

Original Medicare includes two parts: Medicare A and Medicare B. Additionally, parts C and D have been added for other types of coverage. Each part covers a different type of care, and you'll choose how you enroll.

• **Medicare A** covers hospital-based care. If you've worked and paid taxes for at least 10 years,

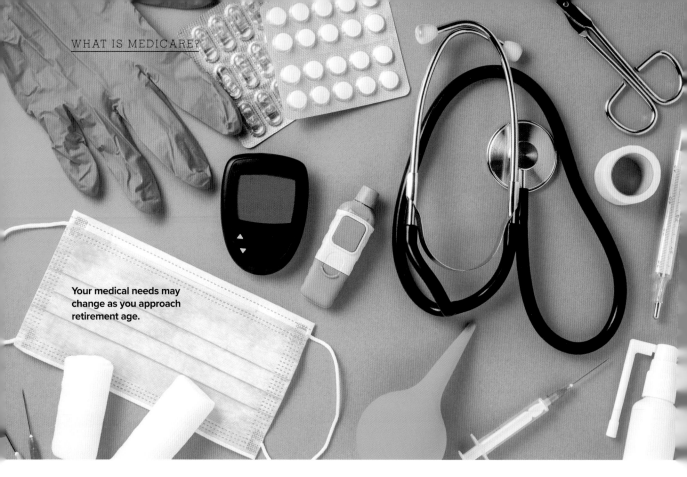

Your medical needs may change as you approach retirement age.

you won't have to pay a monthly premium for Medicare A.

• **Medicare B** covers visits to your doctor's office, outpatient care, preventative services and medical supplies. This part does require a monthly premium, though it's likely to be much less expensive than your previous health insurance.

Educate yourself about how Medicare works before you become eligible, so you know what questions to ask in order to choose the best plan.

• **Medicare C** is a way of bundling parts A, B and usually D. Also known as Medicare Advantage, these plans are offered by Medicare-approved private companies and are often more comprehensive than original Medicare.

• **Medicare D** covers prescription medications.

As you approach eligibility, it's important to educate yourself on the specific ways that Medicare works. Knowing what is available to you and how the different parts all work together will help you ask the right questions, consider your options and choose the right plan, ensuring you have the affordable care you'll need well into the future.

How to Get Medicare

Once you turn 65, you become eligible to take part in Medicare. If you're already collecting Social Security payments when you turn 65, you may be automatically enrolled in parts A and B. If you are not collecting Social Security or disability payments at this point, you'll need to actively enroll. Either way, you'll still want to review all of your options and select the plan that's best for you. ∎

BECOMING AN INFORMED MEDICARE CONSUMER Managing your benefits

While you've heard the word "Medicare" a million times, you may not understand exactly what it is or how it works. Some doctors participate; some don't. The program covers some medical procedures, but not others. Some elected officials praise Medicare, while others are accused of trying to take it apart. Everyone does seem to agree, however, that Medicare is a huge, complicated government program whose intricacies can make your head spin.

The good news is that Medicare serves the needs of a huge pool of beneficiaries across the United States. The downside? It's up to you to make the program work for you. The Department of Health and Human Services will not give you a heads-up when it is time to enroll, and you're responsible for gathering the information that will help you make the best decisions—both before you enroll and once you become a Medicare user.

Start by considering the following list of basic issues and decisions before you get into the more complicated choices. With a little luck, your head will stop spinning and you'll enjoy the peace of

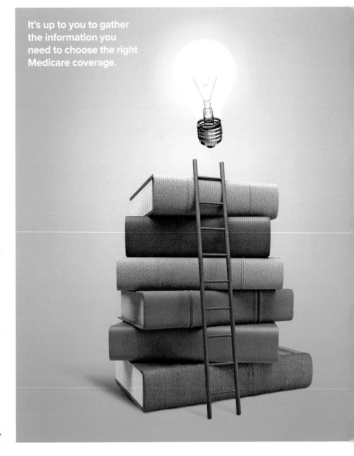

It's up to you to gather the information you need to choose the right Medicare coverage.

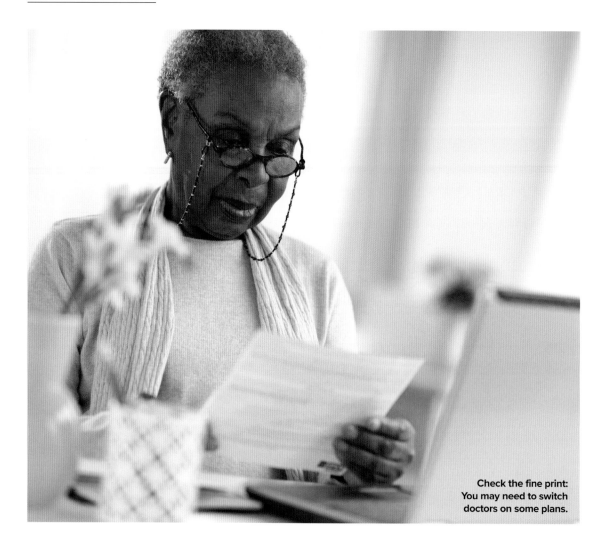

Check the fine print: You may need to switch doctors on some plans.

mind that comes from having the medical coverage that best fits your needs.

•**Get a Basic Understanding of Medicare** You'll need to dive into the details later, but for now, be sure you clearly understand what Medicare Parts A through D cover. It's also important to be clear on the difference between traditional Medicare and its counterpart, Medicare Advantage.

•**Think About Your Personal Situation and the Coverage That You'll Require** Would you be willing to change doctors and/or pharmacies if a certain plan required it? Do you spend significant time at a second home in another state or out of the country? Do you have existing coverage that could augment Medicare? Your answers to these questions are essential to choosing the right Medicare options.

•**Check Your Calendar** Timing is crucial, and it's up to you to know when to enroll. The enrollment window generally opens three months before the month of your 65th birthday and closes seven months later. Although there are a few exceptions, missing the window can be expensive.

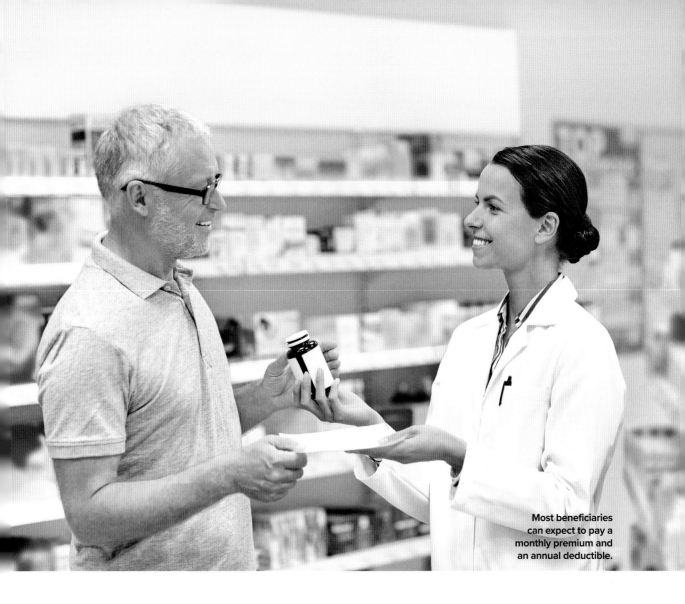

Most beneficiaries can expect to pay a monthly premium and an annual deductible.

• **Understand the Costs** To put it bluntly: Medicare isn't free. Most beneficiaries should expect to pay a monthly premium and some form of deductible for services, though the specifics vary according to your work history and the level of coverage that you select. In many cases, Medicare Advantage premiums are lower than those of traditional Medicare due to the cost-saving effects of bundled coverage.

• **Try Again Next Year** If you don't love the plan you choose initially, you're not wedded to it for life. Whether you participate in tradition-al Medicare or Medicare Advantage, you can change your coverage during the annual election period that runs from Oct. 15 to Dec. 7 each year.

The guide that follows provides a host of information and advice about enrolling in and using Medicare. As you learn how to navigate the system, you may also want to check out the *Medicare & You* handbook available at medicare.gov, or call the toll-free Medicare help line at 800-633-4227. You may also want to check in with your doctor, or with friends and family who have Medicare coverage. ∎

A BRIEF HISTORY OF MEDICARE
This national health-insurance plan was 50 years in the making

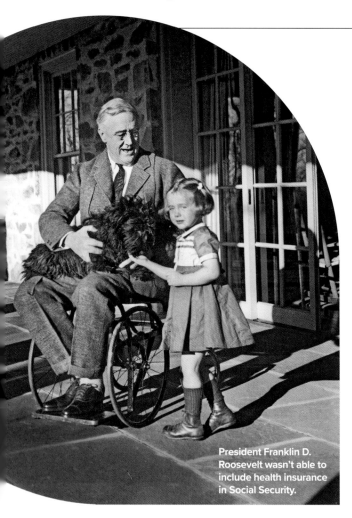

President Franklin D. Roosevelt wasn't able to include health insurance in Social Security.

Medicare didn't become law until 1965, but the program has its roots in a national debate over the government's role in health care that began much earlier. The idea of a national health insurance program goes back at least to Teddy Roosevelt's 1912 Progressive Party campaign for president.

Though medical costs were far lower in Roosevelt's time than they are today, nearly all Americans, apart from a small number of organized laborers, went without insurance. Professional medical organizations actively argued against collectivizing health care costs. Even so, the Progressive platform was popular among working-class Americans eager for access to costly new medical technologies, such as radiography and improved diagnostic tests.

Early Attempts at National Insurance
Roosevelt's defeat at the polls and the opposition of doctors and private business was enough to keep the idea from gaining political traction. Its

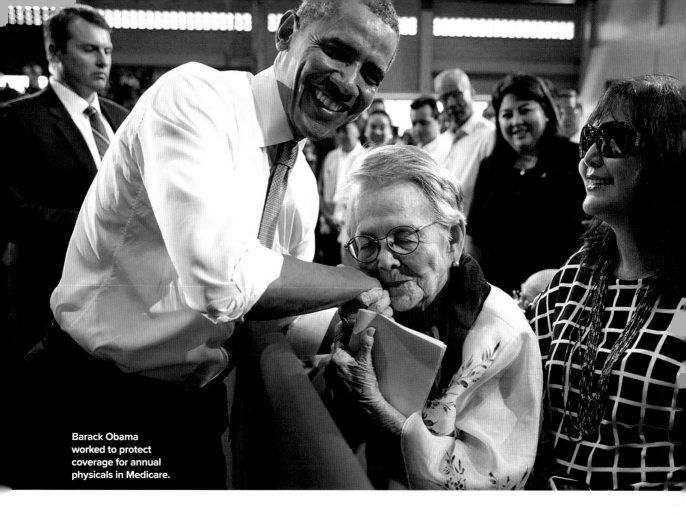

Barack Obama worked to protect coverage for annual physicals in Medicare.

resemblance to Germany's national health program became a political liability when the United States entered World War I. And after Russia's Communist Revolution, ambitious social programs smacked of Bolshevism.

The national health insurance idea was revived in 1935, when President Franklin D. Roosevelt tried, and failed, to include health insurance in his signature Social Security legislation. Ten years later, President Harry S. Truman called on Congress to create a national health insurance fund that would cover all Americans, and a bill was quickly introduced in both chambers. The American Medical Association aggressively lobbied against it, leveraging the widespread fear of communism by branding the effort "socialized medicine." The bill never passed.

Medicare Becomes Law

By the late 1950s, national health insurance was gaining public support. John F. Kennedy narrowly took the White House in 1960 with a campaign platform that included health coverage for Social Security retirees. Kennedy's subsequent effort to enact something like Medicare enjoyed the enthusiastic support of the AFL-CIO. But it drew familiar attacks from the American Medical Association, which took to network television to convince the public they were "in danger of being blitzed, brainwashed and bandwagoned" by Kennedy's proposal. Kennedy's vice president and successor, President Lyndon B. Johnson, capitalized on the momentum of his landslide re-election in 1964 to push a bill through Congress. Medicare was finally signed into law on July 30, 1965, with an initial budget of about $10 billion.

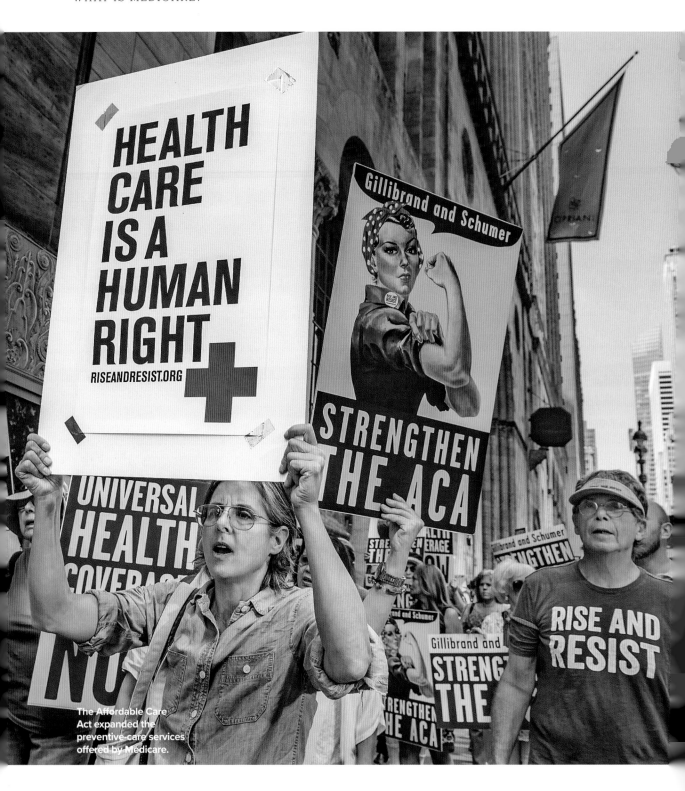

The Affordable Care Act expanded the preventive-care services offered by Medicare.

Besides shifting popular opinion and a recent electoral mandate, Johnson also brought his political acumen to bear in the fight for Medicare. His strategy was to be gentle but relentless in lobbying key Congressional holdouts in his own party. His public message was, "[B]y God, you can't treat Grandma this way. She's entitled and we promised it to her." He likewise appealed to legislators' emotions, telling then-White House assistant Bill Moyers, "[Tell them] that every guy that votes for Medicare and education, his grandchildren will say my grandpa was in the Congress that enacted these two.... So it makes 'em proud."

In the end, the bill passed with bipartisan support, despite having been defeated so many times in previous iterations.

Tweaks and Adjustments

In its original form, Medicare enrolled Americans 65 and older in hospital insurance (Part A). Seniors were invited to sign up for medical insurance (Part B) as well. The first enrollees paid a $3 premium every month, deducted from their Social Security checks, for Part B. At the same time, 0.35 percent of every worker's paycheck was put toward the Medicare system, with employers matching the amount. In its first year, 19 million people signed up for Medicare Part B.

The following year, the Medicare payroll tax rose to 0.5 percent. But the first major change to Medicare came in 1972, when coverage was expanded to include individuals under the age of 65 with long-term disabilities or end-stage renal disease. An omnibus spending bill expanded home health services and brought federal oversight to Medigap—Medicare supplemental insurance—in 1980. In 1986, Congress raised the tax to 1.45 percent (2.9 percent for self-employed workers), where it stands today. Two years later, total out-of-pocket expenses for Part A and Part B were capped by the Medicare Catastrophic Coverage Act. The attendant increase in premiums led to the repeal of most of the law within a

year. In 2013, the government imposed an additional Medicare tax of 0.9 percent for employees with income in excess of $200,000. (The threshold is $250,000 for those married filing jointly.)

The 1990s gave birth to Medicare Part C, originally called Medicare HMOs. The new program offered beneficiaries the option to seek private alternatives to Part A and Part B, known collectively as Original Medicare.

Flawed but Surviving

In 2003, nearly 40 years after Medicare's creation, President George W. Bush signed a bill that created Medicaid Part D, a prescription-drug benefit available through private insurers. In 2010, the Affordable Care Act, known informally as Obamacare, increased Medicare's preventive-care services to include free mammograms, colonoscopies and annual wellness visits. It also sought to improve Part D coverage, raised premiums for some beneficiaries, and authorized an Independent Payment Advisory Board to act as a check on Medicare costs. The board was effectively killed by President Donald Trump. Under his watch, caps on expenses for outpatient therapy have been repealed and coverage has been rolled back for high-income beneficiaries.

Johnson viewed the original Medicare legislation as flawed. He conceded privately, for example, that the bill had too few cost controls. His attitude was that any problems "can be fixed once it sinks in that Medicare is here to stay." His instincts have mostly been borne out. Today, nearly 60 million Americans receive insurance through Medicare. The program is popular with a majority of Americans, regardless of political affiliation, even as two-thirds of them believe it could use some changes. ∎

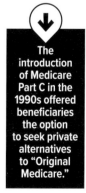

The introduction of Medicare Part C in the 1990s offered beneficiaries the option to seek private alternatives to "Original Medicare."

SENIOR HEALTH CARE SYSTEMS AROUND THE WORLD How Medicare compares

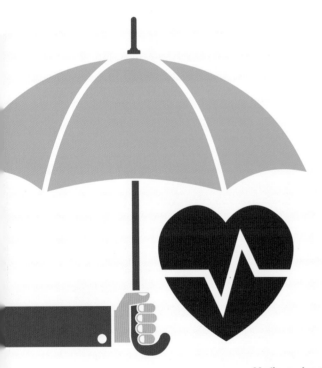

Medicare aims to ensure U.S. citizens have medical coverage during retirement.

Your retirement is supposed to be your golden years, when you can enjoy the fruits of your labor, kick back and relax. Yet it's also when many people leave their jobs—and the health insurance benefits many employers provide. In the United States, Medicare aims to cover that gap and ensure that people have medical coverage even as they age.

In 2020, Medicare covers 62 million people age 65 or older. Medicare is a single-payer system, meaning it is provided by one entity—the federal government—and is financed by payroll taxes as well as the individuals who receive it.

Although coverage is universal for seniors, most Americans don't have government-backed health insurance. According to the U.S. Census Bureau, the majority of Americans (55 percent) got health insurance through their jobs in 2018, while 18 percent of the population received Medicaid—a program jointly funded by the federal government and states to provide health coverage for low-income and disabled individuals. Those without access to employer-sponsored health insurance and who do not qualify for ei-

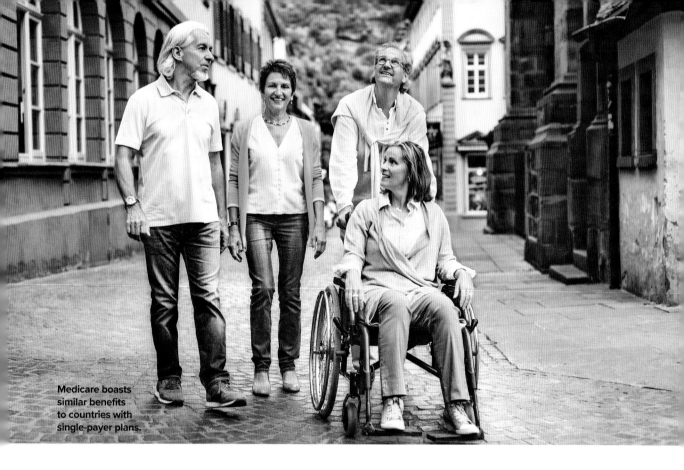

Medicare boasts similar benefits to countries with single-payer plans.

ther Medicare or Medicaid can purchase individual private plans.

When it comes to health care around the world, the United States is an outlier. All other developed countries provide some level of universal health coverage for all their citizens, whereas the U.S. federal government only provides coverage for people over 65.

Health Care Systems Around the World

The countries that provide universal coverage tend to adopt one of three models:

• **Single-Payer** In countries with single-payer systems, national, regional or local governments pay for health care by taxing citizens. Countries with this model include Canada, the United Kingdom and Sweden. Even within this model, there are some differences in how insurance operates. The U.K., for instance, provides single-payer socialized medicine through its National Health Service, in which the government both pays for and provides medical services. In Canada, however, the government finances health care costs, while the private sector delivers the services. Many Canadians purchase supplemental private insurance policies to cover services not included in the national plan, such as optometry and dental care.

• **Insurance Mandate** This method requires citizens to purchase insurance through private, public or nonprofit insurers. Germany uses this system. While the majority of Germans get their coverage through the national public system, others opt to purchase private health insurance. Private insurance options are particularly attractive for young

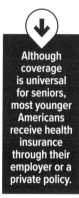

Although coverage is universal for seniors, most younger Americans receive health insurance through their employer or a private policy.

19

people with solid incomes because insurers may offer them a wider range of services and lower premiums. No federal subsidies exist for private insurance, but the government does regulate premiums, and cost-sharing is capped for low-income people and reduced for those with chronic illnesses.

• **Two-Tiered Approach** With a two-tiered approach, the government taxes its citizens to pay for basic health services, while allowing the option to supplement with private insurance. France is one example of a two-tier system: Its mandatory public insurance covers 70 to 80 percent of costs, while voluntary private health insurance picks up the rest (or citizens end up paying out of pocket).

How Medicare Compares

Because Medicare operates as a single-payer system, it boasts similar benefits as those associated with other countries' single-payer plans, such as lower administrative costs and higher rates of coverage among seniors. However, out-of-pocket expenses associated with Medicare, such as premium contributions and cost-sharing, add a financial barrier for seniors accessing care. By contrast, Canada and the United Kingdom require no deductibles or cost-sharing for any primary-care services. Meanwhile, in Sweden most elderly care is funded by municipal taxes and government grants, while seniors' remaining health care costs are largely subsidized.

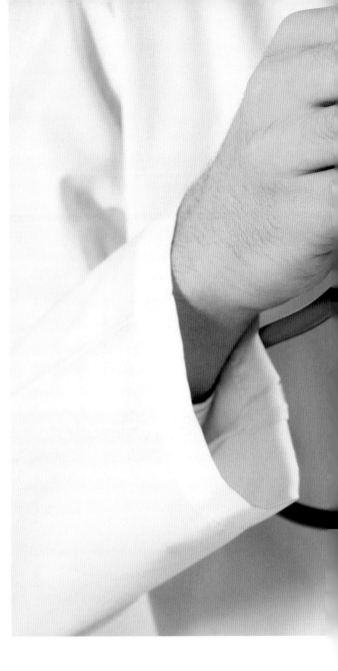

U.S. seniors are more likely to skip or delay medical treatment due to high costs than those in other developed countries, according to a 2017 survey.

As a result, seniors in the U.S. are more likely to skip or delay medical treatment due to high costs, according to a 2017 survey by the Commonwealth Fund. The survey compared the population of adults 65 and older in the U.S., Australia, Canada, France, Germany, the Netherlands, Norway, Sweden, Switzerland and the United Kingdom. Twenty-three percent of U.S. respondents said they had skipped recommended medical tests or treatments, delayed seeing a doctor when sick or skipped filling a prescription in 2016 due to the high costs associated with these services. Just 5 percent or fewer respondents in the U.K., France, Norway and Sweden reported skipping services due to cost.

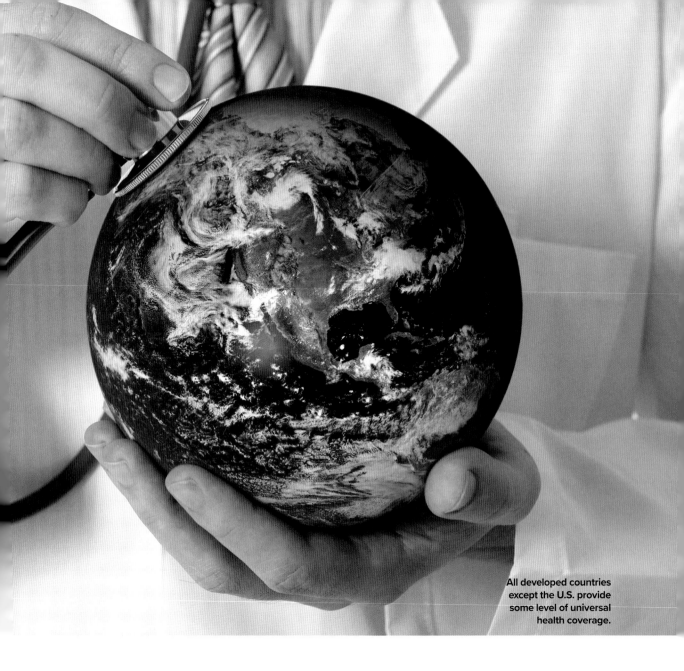

All developed countries except the U.S. provide some level of universal health coverage.

When it comes to out-of-pocket expenses, the U.S. and Switzerland are outliers compared to the other countries in the survey. Nearly one in four U.S. seniors (22 percent) and one of three Swiss respondents (31 percent) reported spending $2,000 or more in out-of-pocket costs, such as coinsurance, prescription drugs and copays. Fewer than 10 percent of seniors in other countries reported spending as much.

Despite the challenges rising medical costs pose to Medicare, the program has achieved its goal of expanding coverage to seniors, giving older Americans an option for coverage in retirement. Before Medicare was established, 48 percent of adults 65 and older were uninsured. Today, only 2 percent of adults age 65 and older are uninsured, meaning more seniors are covered as they age. ∎

THE CURRENT MEDICARE DEBATE
Understanding the political tug-of-war

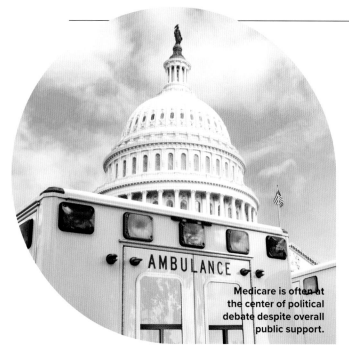

Medicare is often at the center of political debate despite overall public support.

Even the casual political observer can't help but notice that Medicare, along with other "entitlement" programs, seems to be constantly on the chopping block in the halls of Washington, D.C. That makes sense, as Medicare is an ideological lightning rod. Conservatives believe the system is a money-waster that would be more efficient if it were privatized, while liberals see it as a key element of a robust social-welfare system.

That political tug-of-war is complicated by the fact that the program is broadly popular among Americans. Even most self-identified Republicans said that the government "should continue programs like Medicare and Medicaid" in a 2017 Pew Research poll. Meanwhile, a Kaiser Family Foundation poll from January 2019 found that 77 percent of Americans would like to see Medicare expanded to allow people between the ages of 50 and 64 to buy into the system. Politicians from either side of the ideological divide have always sold pushes for reform as "preserving" Medicare, whatever the content of the proposal.

In fact, the idea of a publicly funded national health insurance program has inspired activism and opposition since it was first taken up by Teddy Roosevelt's Progressive Party in 1912. And the eventual passage of Medicare legislation in 1965 came after a heated debate that saw the American Medical Association derisively cast it as "socialized medicine," while Ronald Reagan, who had recently switched to the Republican party, warned that Medicare's passage would imperil "every area of freedom as we have known it in this country." Proponents of the system likewise couched their argument in emotionally intense terms, painting Medicare as the least that was owed to "grandma."

The Drug Pricing Debate

Today, much of the Medicare debate concerns prescription drug pricing. Everyone seems to agree that prescription drugs cost far too much in the United States, but solutions usually differ between political parties. A Democratic proposal would have empowered Medicare to set lower prices for brand-name drugs for its beneficiaries. If the manufacturer refused, the government could allow another company to produce a generic version.

Republicans initially dismissed the plan as socialism. However, President Donald Trump, who occasionally defies conservative orthodoxy, embraced the historically liberal position in 2018. Some Republicans have since followed suit, backing proposals that would give the government greater power to set drug prices or reimport medicines from Canada at a lower cost. If that shift holds, it's possible that the government may make some progress on lowering drug prices, whether or not that approach satisfies the pharmaceuticals industry.

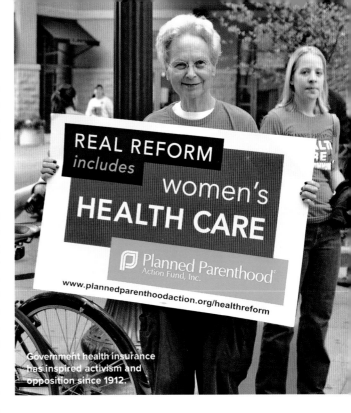

Government health insurance has inspired activism and opposition since 1912.

Funding Medicare's Future

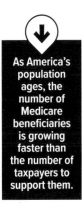

As America's population ages, the number of Medicare beneficiaries is growing faster than the number of taxpayers to support them.

Another perennial source of debate is Medicare's uncertain financial future. The program, which was never self-financing, will likely become more expensive in the future. Medicare's Hospital Insurance trust fund, which pays for Part A benefits, is expected to be drained by 2026. That will create a funding gap, as dedicated revenues will only cover 89 percent of Medicare hospital insurance costs. The Supplementary Medical Insurance trust fund, which pays for Part B and Part D benefits, can't be depleted per se: Its premiums and other revenues are set according to Medicare users' actual costs. Even so, it's getting costlier. America's aging population means the increase in Medicare beneficiaries is outpacing the increase in workers paying taxes to support them.

Republicans prefer solving the problem through privatization and consumer choice. A common proposal is to increase the use of medical savings accounts, which the beneficiary would use to pay deductibles on qualified medical expenses. Democrats are more likely to support raising taxes to keep benefits in place.

As long as Medicare remains broadly popular among American voters, it would be hard for either party to dismantle it or drastically change what's covered. But meanwhile, conservatives will look for ways to increasingly privatize the program and liberals will continue to advocating for more public funding. ∎

MEDICARE MYTHS Check your knowledge against these common misconceptions

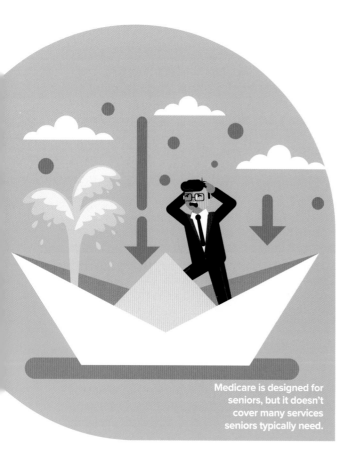

Medicare is designed for seniors, but it doesn't cover many services seniors typically need.

MYTH NO. 1
Medicare Is Free

Reality: While Medicare should significantly decrease your health care costs, it's not completely free. Even if you don't pay a premium for Part A, you'll still pay a deductible and coinsurance charges. Besides those fees, you'll pay a premium for Parts B and D, as well as for any Medigap or Medicare Advantage plan you choose.

MYTH NO. 2
Medicare Is Going Broke

Reality: This isn't totally a myth, but it's not completely true, either. The latest reports from the Medicare Trustees—who oversee the fund that covers Part A—say that by 2026, the fund won't be able to cover its costs. While that conclusion may worry those approaching retirement, it's still possible for Congress to create a budget that protects Medicare benefits while keeping the fund solvent. What's more, Parts B and D are not affected by the fund's shortfall, which means that much of the Medicare system can continue to pay for itself.

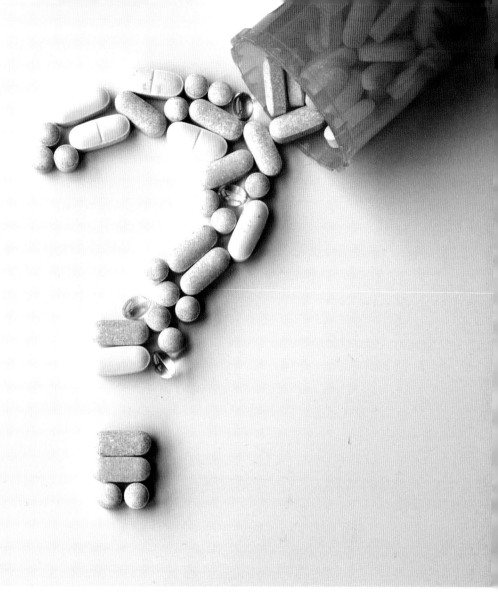

Not all types of Medicare cover prescription medications.

You'll Be Enrolled Automatically

Reality: Most people have to actively enroll in Medicare. The government will not automatically enroll you or send you a reminder to enroll. But there are exceptions. For instance, people already receiving benefits through Social Security will be automatically enrolled in Parts A and B. However, if you're in this group, you'll still need to actively enroll in Part D and decide whether you want to also enroll in Medigap coverage or a Medicare Advantage plan.

Medicare Covers Everything

Reality: Even though Medicare is designed for seniors, it doesn't cover certain services, including vision, hearing and dental care. And although Medicare does cover care in a "skilled nursing facility," that coverage is limited to short-term, medically necessary stays. It does not include long-term care in a nursing home or assisted-living facility. You may want to look into other sources of funding, such as long-term care insurance, to cover those expenses. ∎

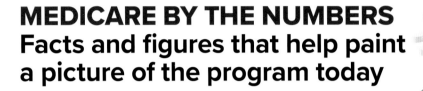

MEDICARE BY THE NUMBERS
Facts and figures that help paint a picture of the program today

1965
The year President Lyndon Johnson signed Medicare into law under Title XVIII of the Social Security Act.

1972
The year President Richard Nixon expanded Medicare to include people under age 65 who have long-term disabilities or end-stage renal disease.

62 million
Approximate number of people now enrolled in Medicare.

$731 billion
Total Medicare benefit payments in 2018. Of that, 32 percent was spent by Medicare Advantage plans, and 13 percent covered Medicare Part D.

$144.60
2020 standard monthly premium for Medicare Part B, which covers physician visits and outpatient services.

$198
2020 Medicare Part B annual deductible.

22 million
Number of people enrolled in Medicare Advantage in 2019, up from 10.5 million in 2009.

47 million
Number of people enrolled in Medicare Part D, which provides outpatient prescription drug benefits, in 2020. That's more than 75 percent of all Medicare enrollees.

67%
Percentage of Medicare Advantage enrollees who had dental benefits through their coverage in 2019. Among the same population, 72 percent had fitness benefits and 78 percent had eye-care benefits.

2026
The year through which Medicare will remain solvent, or able to pay 100 percent of the costs of the hospital insurance it provides. ∎

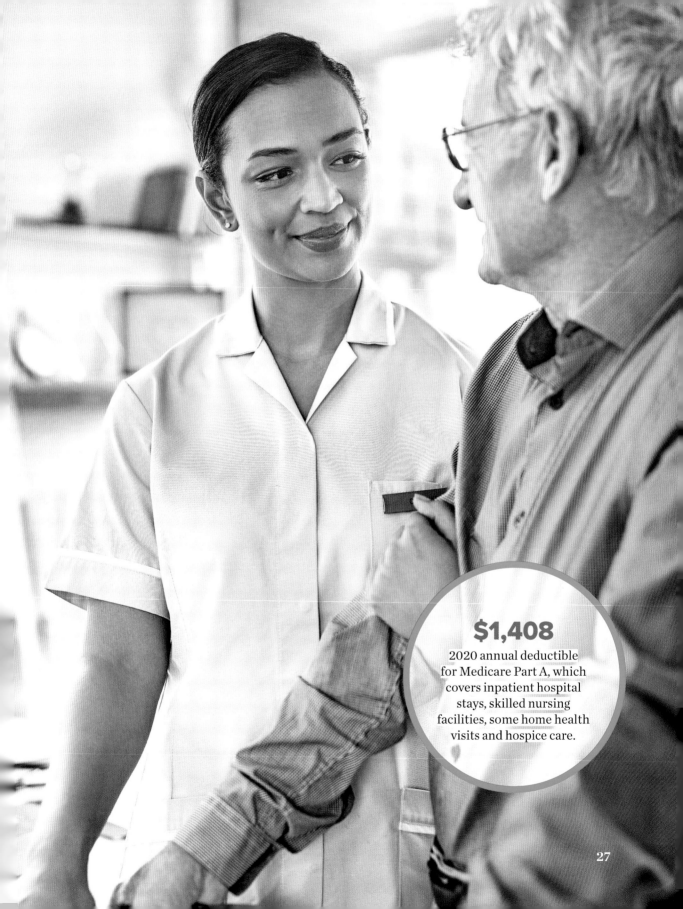

$1,408

2020 annual deductible for Medicare Part A, which covers inpatient hospital stays, skilled nursing facilities, some home health visits and hospice care.

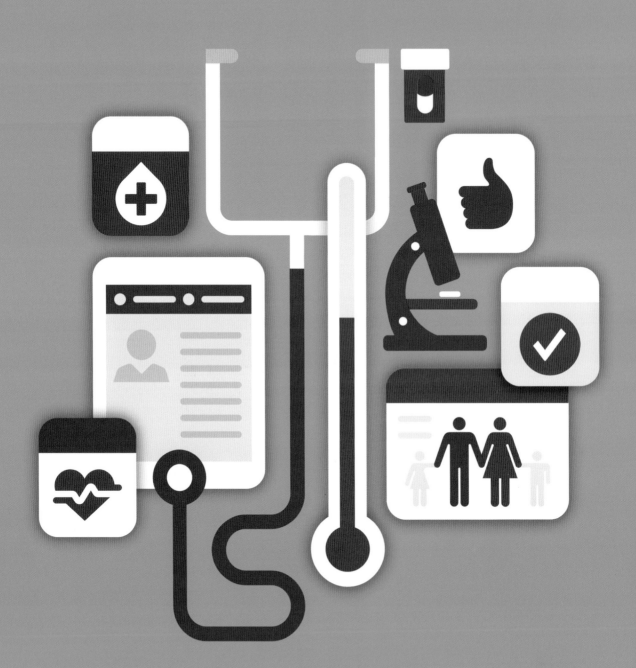

Getting Medicare

Information and tips for when and how to enroll

WHAT YOU NEED TO KNOW ABOUT ELIGIBILITY There's more to it than how many candles are on your cake

Most people become eligible for Medicare when they turn 65. However, becoming eligible doesn't mean you're automatically enrolled or that all of your health care needs are covered. It simply means that you're allowed to sign up. But what you're eligible for, when you sign up and where you live will all factor into the type of plan you end up with—and how much it costs.

Eligibility at 65

Not all of us look forward to our birthday. But if you're about to turn 65, you absolutely have something to look forward to: eligibility for Medicare. When you turn 65, you'll be automatically eligible as long as you're a U.S. citizen or legal resident and have lived in the United States constantly for at least five years.

To qualify for premium-free Part A, you'll have to meet at least one of the following requirements:

• You are eligible for Social Security (generally, this means you've worked and paid Medicare taxes for at least 10 years).

• Your spouse has worked and paid Medicare taxes for at least 10 years and is at least 62 years old.

• You or your spouse is a current or retired government employee who has paid Medicare payroll taxes during their career.

• You or your spouse qualifies for retirement benefits through the Railroad Retirement Board.

If you're divorced or your spouse is deceased (and you haven't remarried), you may also qualify for premium-free or reduced-premium Part A based on your spouse or former spouse's work history. So even if you haven't worked, your former spouse's credits may exempt you from paying a premium for Part A. However, there are restrictions: To qualify for premium-free Part A based on a former spouse's work history, you must have been married for at least 10 years. To qualify based on a deceased

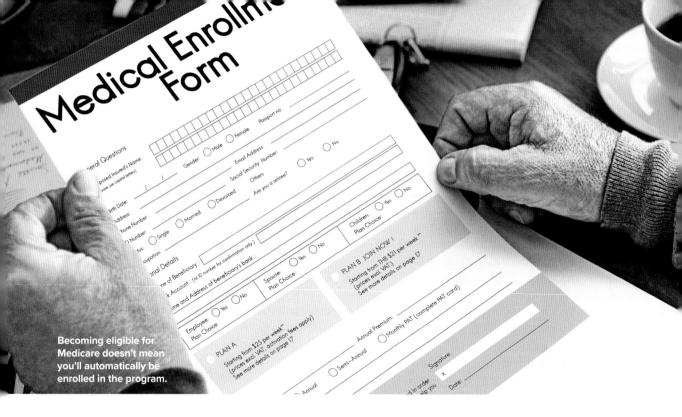

Medical Enrollment Form

Becoming eligible for Medicare doesn't mean you'll automatically be enrolled in the program.

spouse's work history, you must have been married for at least nine months prior to his or her death.

It's also important to note that unlike private health insurance plans, Medicare is intended strictly for individuals. You cannot add dependents such as children onto your Medicare plan. Even eligible spouses must enroll on their own.

When You're Eligible to Sign Up

You become eligible to enroll in Medicare three months before your 65th birthday. At that point, the government gives you a seven-month window during which you are able to sign up for Parts A and B.

This seven-month window, known as your initial enrollment period (IEP), includes:

• The three months before your 65th birthday

• The month of your 65th birthday

• The three months after your 65th birthday

Generally, you'll want to sign up for Part A as soon as you're eligible, since your coverage will begin based on when you enroll. If you don't sign up during this period, you'll pay a late penalty. You also won't be able to enroll until the next general enrollment period, which lasts from Jan. 1 through March 31. That coverage begins July 1.

If you're still working and have private insurance through your employer, you can enroll in Part A and delay signing up for Part B until you're no longer working. This approach lets you put off paying the Part B premium until you retire. However, if you work for a company with fewer than 20 employees you don't have this option. In that case, Medicare will become your primary insurer as soon as you turn 65, which means you'll need to sign up for Part B.

Eligibility Before 65

People with certain qualifying disabilities and illnesses are eligible for Medicare before they

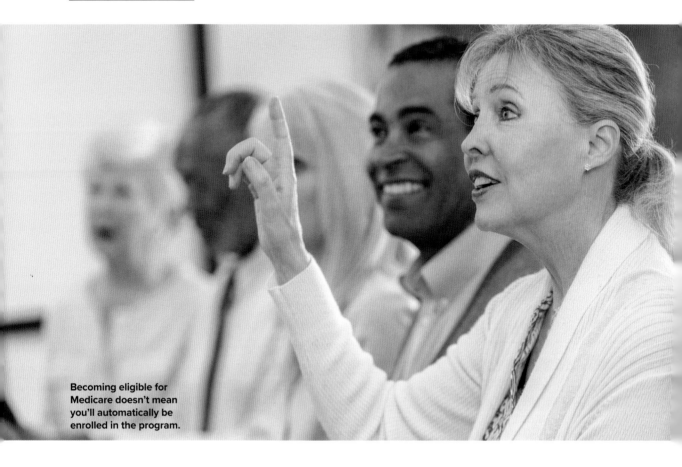

Becoming eligible for Medicare doesn't mean you'll automatically be enrolled in the program.

turn 65. Some people qualify for Medicare regardless of age, including the following:

• People who have been receiving Social Security Disability Insurance (SSDI) benefits for at least 24 months

• People with ALS (also known as Lou Gehrig's disease)

• People with end-stage renal disease (ESRD)

Eligibility Beyond Part A

Once you become eligible for Part A, you also automatically become eligible for the oth-

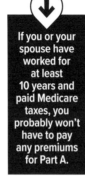

If you or your spouse have worked for at least 10 years and paid Medicare taxes, you probably won't have to pay any premiums for Part A.

er parts of Medicare, including Parts B and D, Medigap and Medicare Advantage. However, each of these additional parts comes with its own costs. Those who can't afford these costs may also be eligible for Medicaid—the government program that provides health insurance for low-income people.

Unlike Medicare, Medicaid is administered by states, so the qualifications will depend on where you live. If you do qualify for Medicaid, it is possible to carry both Medicare and Medicaid simultaneously. In fact, about one in five Medicare recipients is also on Medicaid. Even if you're not eligible for full Medicaid coverage, you may qualify for a Medicare Savings Program. These programs are based on your income level and can help keep your health care costs affordable. ∎

PAYING FOR MEDICARE: AN OVERVIEW
There are many ways to pay, so choose the one that works for you

Paying for Original Medicare

"Original Medicare" includes Parts A and B. Since these two parts are administered by the federal government, you'll pay Medicare directly for your Part B premium (and your Part A premium, if you have one). There are multiple ways to set up your payments:

• If you're already receiving retirement benefits though Social Security or the Railroad Retirement Board, your premium will be automatically deducted from your benefits payment.

• You can sign up for Medicare Easy Pay, a free online system that allows Medicare to automatically deduct your premiums from your bank account. To sign up, you'll need to mail in a form and wait six to eight weeks for processing.

• Alternatively, many banks allow customers to set up automated bill pay. This connects your bank with your Medicare bill, so that your bank can automatically make the payments from your checking account each period.

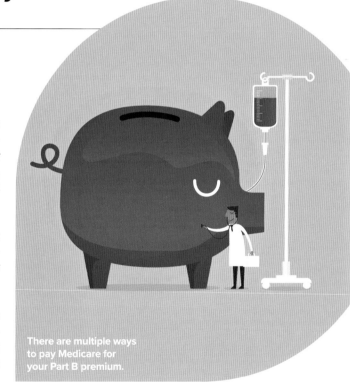

There are multiple ways to pay Medicare for your Part B premium.

• Manual payments can also be made with a check, money order, debit card or credit card. This approach allows you to pay your bill without automating payments.

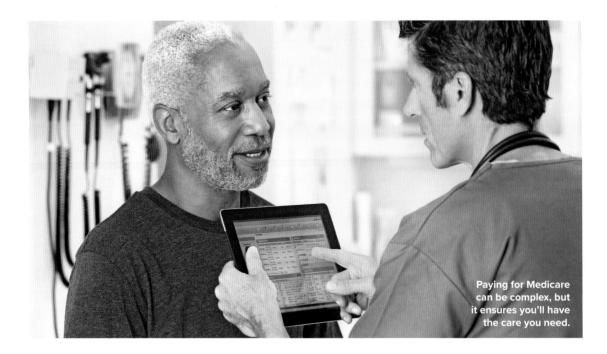

Paying for Medicare can be complex, but it ensures you'll have the care you need.

Federal retirees who don't receive Social Security but receive an annuity from the Office of Personnel Management won't have their premiums automatically deducted from their annuity payments. However, they may request automatic deductions through Medicare.

When Your Payment Isn't Taken Out of Social Security

If you aren't yet receiving retirement benefits through Social Security, Medicare will send you a bill for your premium. This bill is form CMS-500. It will list the dates that your payment will cover (generally the following three months). If you missed a payment or have had a change in your premium amount, your bill will reflect that, too. In most cases, you'll receive your bill on or around the 10th of each month. Payment is due by the

Medicare will send you a bill for your premium every three months, but you'll also have a three-month grace period to make your payment.

25th. Medicare bills quarterly, so you can expect a bill every three months. However, if paying for an entire quarter at once creates a financial hardship, you can contact your local Social Security office to ask for monthly bills instead.

Though the due date for your bill will be the 25th of the month, Medicare offers a three-month grace period for you to make your payment. Once this grace period expires, you'll receive two notices in the mail reminding you to pay, after which Medicare can cancel your enrollment in Part B. If your Part B coverage is canceled, you'll need to re-enroll during the next open enrollment period, and your coverage won't begin again for a couple of months after that. You could also face permanent late-enrollment charges, potentially increasing your premium for the rest of your life.

Paying for Part D

If your income is below $87,000 per year (or $174,000 jointly), you can simply pay your Medicare Part D premium directly to the private insur-

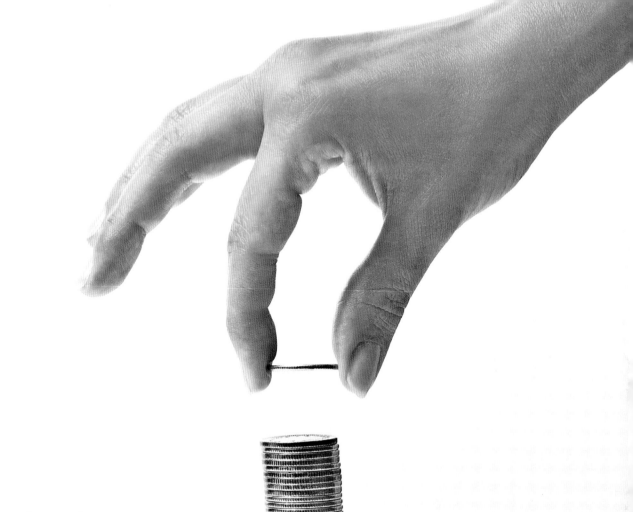

Medicare premiums can add up, so be sure to select options that work for your budget.

er that issued the policy. If your income exceeds that level, though, you may be required to pay a Part D Income Related Monthly Adjustment Amount (Part D-IRMAA). If you are required to pay a Part D-IRMAA, you'll make that payment directly to Medicare while paying your monthly premium to your Part D plan.

And don't forget about the IRMAA—if you fail to pay it, you can lose your Part D coverage and might not be able to get it back. To make things simpler, you can have your Part D premium automatically deducted from your Social Security check, but you'll have to contact your plan (not the Social Security office) to arrange that.

Paying for Medigap and Medicare Advantage

If you enroll in a Medigap plan, you'll pay your Medigap premium to your Medigap insurer—not to Medicare. Likewise, if you opt for Medicare Advantage, you'll pay any related premium to the plan's private insurer. It is possible to have those premiums automatically deducted from your benefits check, but you'll have to contact the Social Security office to arrange that. ■

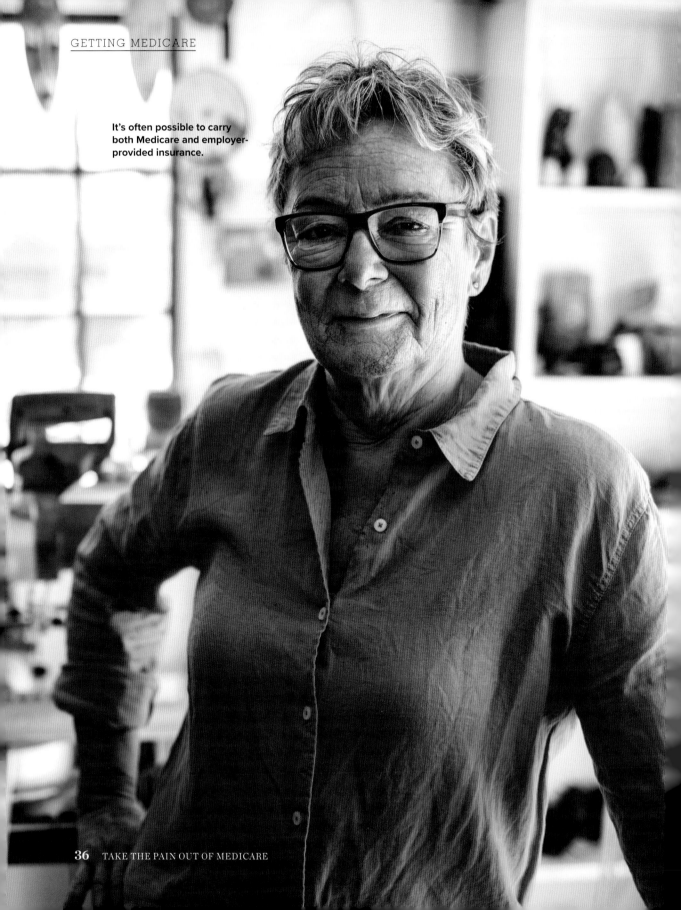

It's often possible to carry both Medicare and employer-provided insurance.

GETTING MEDICARE WHEN YOU'RE STILL WORKING Even if you're still on the job, don't let your initial enrollment period pass you by

Today, it's fairly common to work beyond the age of 65. People are living longer, healthier lives, so many are putting off retirement as a way to continue building their savings and collecting workplace benefits. While there is a financial incentive to wait until full retirement age to collect Social Security benefits, it's best for most people to sign up for Medicare as soon as they're eligible. In many cases, it's possible to carry both Medicare and private insurance, so enrolling doesn't have to mean losing the coverage you already have.

Note that the following information refers to those still actively working. If you've stopped working but have COBRA when you become eligible for Medicare, your COBRA coverage will end and you need to enroll in Medicare promptly.

Signing Up for Part A

Part A is the most basic aspect of Medicare, covering hospital-related costs. If you've already earned your 40 work credits—meaning you've paid at least 10 years' worth of Medicare taxes—you'll get this part without having to pay any monthly premium.

Because Part A doesn't cost anything, even people who are still covered by an employer's insurance plan should sign up during their Individual Enrollment Period (IEP). That's the seven-month period that begins three months before your 65th birthday. Once your Medicare Part A goes into effect, you'll have a kind of dual coverage: Any hospital-related care will be covered by your private insurance first, with Medicare kicking in second.

Though most people will benefit from enrolling in Part A as soon as they're eligible, there are two big exceptions:

The first is if you have a health savings account (HSA). If you have an HSA, neither you nor your employer are allowed to continue contributing to it

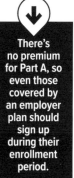

There's no premium for Part A, so even those covered by an employer plan should sign up during their enrollment period.

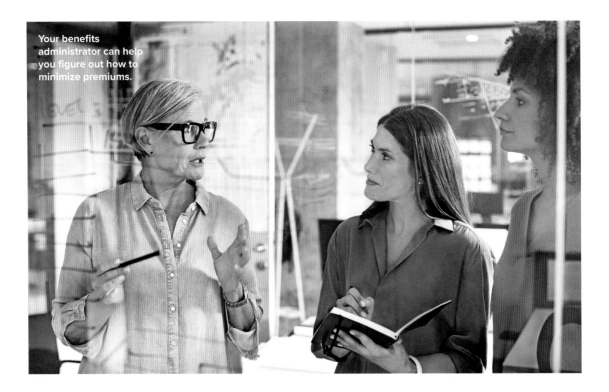

Your benefits administrator can help you figure out how to minimize premiums.

once you've enrolled in Medicare. Therefore, if you want to squeeze in a few more years of HSA savings, it may be in your best interest to put off enrolling in Part A.

However, be aware that the IRS will charge you a tax penalty if you enroll in Part A more than six months after turning 65. When you enroll, the IRS will consider you retroactively enrolled for the previous six months—meaning you'll have to pay taxes on any HSA contributions that you made during that time. To avoid this situation, make sure you stop contributing to your HSA six months before you enroll in Part A.

The second exception is if you don't qualify for premium-free Part A. If you haven't earned your 40 work credits (and can't claim them through a spouse), you'll pay a premium for Part A. If you're currently working to earn those credits, you'll save money by waiting to sign up until you qualify for premium-free Part A.

Signing Up for Part B

Part B always has a premium. For most people, it's $144.60 per month. But if you get insurance through an employer with more than 20 employees, Medicare will allow you to delay enrolling in Part B without any kind of penalty—even if you get the insurance through your spouse.

If your employer has fewer than 20 employees, you will need to enroll in Part B during your IEP. You'll be able to keep your employer's insurance plan as well, but Medicare will become your primary insurer—covering costs before your private insurance plan takes effect.

If you wish to delay enrolling in Part B, talk to your benefits administrator to determine when you should enroll. Some private insurance plans require you to sign up for Parts A and B to get full coverage through their plan. Your benefits administrator can help you understand how Medicare will interact with your current plan, how to

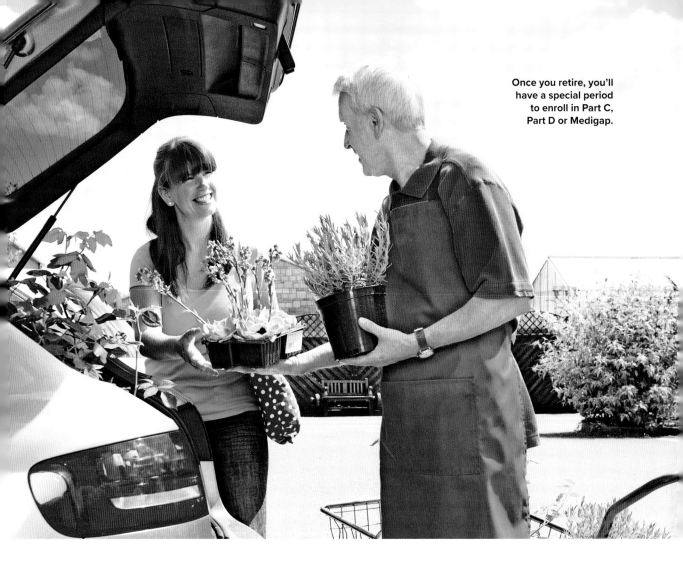

Once you retire, you'll have a special period to enroll in Part C, Part D or Medigap.

minimize premium costs and how to make sure you're never without coverage.

Keep in mind that Medicare will automatically enroll you in Parts A and B once you turn 65 if you collect Social Security—even if you're still working. In that case, you'll have to contact the Social Security office to avoid automatic enrollment in Part B.

Part D, Medicare Advantage and Medigap
Once you're no longer covered by employer insurance, Medicare grants you a special enrollment period (SEP) for Part D, Medigap and Medicare Advantage. During this time, insurers cannot deny you coverage or charge you extra based on your age or medical history. However, once your SEP is over, there is no guarantee that a private insurer will cover you.

For Part D and Medicare Advantage, your SEP lasts for two months after the month your private coverage ends. For Medigap, the open enrollment lasts for six months and begins when you enroll in Part B. ■

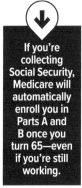

If you're collecting Social Security, Medicare will automatically enroll you in Parts A and B once you turn 65—even if you're still working.

HOW TO ENROLL IN MEDICARE
With multiple ways to sign up, it doesn't have to be a headache

Some people don't have to do anything to sign up for Original Medicare: If you're already collecting retirement benefits through Social Security or the Railroad Retirement Board four months before you turn 65, you'll be automatically enrolled. However, if you haven't yet started collecting these benefits, you'll have to gather some original documents—and a little patience.

How to Enroll
If you're not automatically enrolled in Original Medicare, you have three options for signing up. If you want to enroll over the phone, you'll need to call 800-772-1213 (TTY 800-325-0778). When you do, you'll be able to schedule a phone interview, during which you can formally apply for Medicare.

If you're more comfortable applying in person, you can go to your local Social Security office for an in-person interview. To avoid waiting in line, you can even call ahead and schedule an appointment.

If your 65th birthday is less than three months away, you can also apply online via the Social Security website. However, online applications are only for people who live inside the U.S., don't already have any Medicare coverage, and don't need to apply for retirement benefits at the same time.

Necessary Documents
When you apply for Medicare, you'll need to provide the following:

• Your Social Security number

• Your original birth certificate or a certified copy

• Legal residency documents, such as a passport or green card

• Your marital status; if you're married, you'll need your original marriage certificate or a certified copy

• Proof of your employer-sponsored insurance policy, if you delayed signing up for Part B

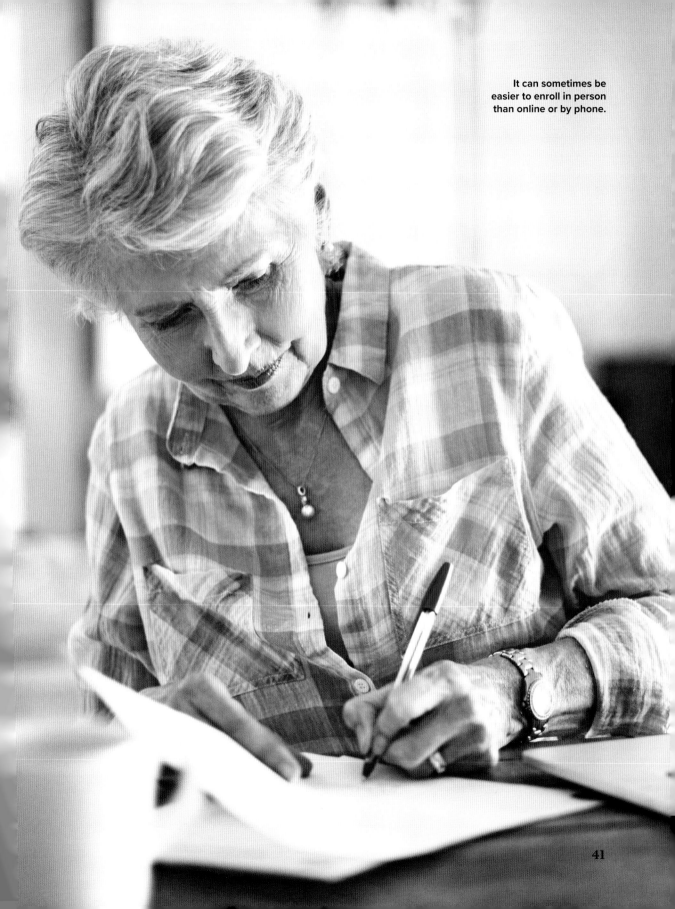

It can sometimes be easier to enroll in person than online or by phone.

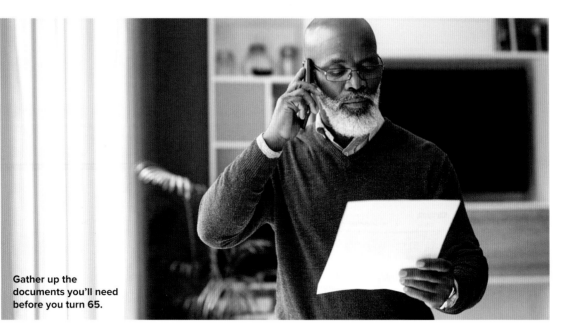

Gather up the documents you'll need before you turn 65.

Because Medicare requires original documents or certified copies, those applying by phone or online will need to mail their documents to Social Security. Regular photocopies are not acceptable. As a result, many people prefer to enroll in person, to keep their documents from getting lost or damaged in transit. If you're a legal resident of the United States and hold a green card, Social Security requests that you apply in person to avoid mailing foreign documents and immigration papers, which can be especially difficult to replace if lost.

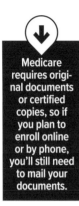

Medicare requires original documents or certified copies, so if you plan to enroll online or by phone, you'll still need to mail your documents.

Though enrolling online or over the phone may seem like less hassle than a potentially long wait at the Social Security office, many people find an in-person interview to be the best of the three methods. In addition to keeping your papers out of the mail, it allows you to spend time with a real person who can answer your questions, look over your spe-cific situation and make sure you understand the details of your potential plan.

Enrolling Under Age 65

Those under 65 with disabilities will be automatically enrolled in Parts A and B after they've received Social Security Disability Insurance (SSDI) benefits for 24 months. If you've been diagnosed with amyotrophic lateral sclerosis (ALS, aka Lou Gehrig's disease), you'll be automatically enrolled in Medicare the first month that you receive your SSDI benefits, which should be five months after you apply. To ensure this happens, be sure that your SSDI application clearly states that you have been diagnosed with ALS.

Those with end-stage renal disease (ESRD) must apply in person at their local Social Security office. Your doctor or dialysis center will give you documentation proving you're eligible for Medicare. If you are too sick to go to the office in person, a family member or other designee can go in your place. ∎

WHEN TO SIGN UP FOR MEDICARE
If you're not automatically enrolled, you'll need to keep track of deadlines—and understand what happens if you miss them

Medicare has strict rules about what types of coverage you can sign up for and when you can sign up for them. Figuring out the deadlines can be complicated, so it's important to consider your situation and work out the enrollment period that works best for you.

Initial Enrollment Period
During your initial enrollment period (IEP), you can sign up for Medicare Parts A and B, as well as Medicare Advantage, Medigap and Part D. To calculate your IEP, start with the month you turn 65. The initial enrollment period lasts seven months, beginning three months before the month of your birthday and ending three months afterward. In other words, if you turn 65 on May 4, your IEP begins Feb. 1 and lasts until Aug. 31 of that year.

For most people, the IEP is the most advantageous time to enroll. If you sign up during the first three months of the period, you can guarantee that your coverage will go into effect as soon as you turn 65.

Special Enrollment Period
If you're still working and covered by employer-based insurance, you may want to delay signing up for Part B, since you don't need full coverage through Medicare yet. If your employer has more than 20 employees, Medicare will grant you a special enrollment period (SEP), during which you can enroll in Part B at the regular premium. This arrangement allows you to avoid the penalty you would otherwise face for delaying your Part B enrollment.

The SEP begins when your IEP ends and continues until eight months after you stop working or lose your employer-sponsored coverage. The eight-month window begins on the first of the month after you lose coverage or stop working, so if you retire on June 18, your eight-month

SEP begins July 1 and lasts until the end of the following February. SEPs also apply if you get your insurance through your spouse's employer, even if you're not working.

You can delay enrollment in a Medicare Advantage Plan or Part D for similar reasons. You'll have to move more quickly, though—the SEP for those plans lasts only 63 days after you lose your employer's coverage.

General Enrollment Period

If you fail to enroll in Parts A and B during your IEP or SEP, you can still enroll during the annual general enrollment period (GEP), which lasts from Jan. 1 to March 31 of each year. If you sign up during this period, your coverage will take effect July 1. You'll also pay higher premiums unless you qualify for premium-free Part A coverage, in which case you'll only pay more for Part B.

Open Enrollment Period

If you don't sign up for Medicare Advantage or Part D during your IEP or SEP, you'll need to wait until the next open enrollment period (OEP), which lasts from Oct. 15 to Dec. 7 each year. If you enroll during this period, your coverage will begin Jan. 1. It's important to note that the OEP and the GEP take place at different times of the year and apply to different Medicare coverages, so you'll need to make sure you pick the appropriate one based on the type of coverage you want.

Medigap

Once you enroll in Part B (whether during your IEP, SEP or open enrollment), you have six months during which you can enroll in a Medigap plan without being denied coverage or overcharged based on age or medical history. This six-month period begins as soon as you enroll in Part B and cannot be postponed. If you're hoping to enroll in Medigap, watch the calendar to avoid being locked out. (For more details on Medigap, see page 61.)

Penalties for Late Enrollment

Missing the Medicare enrollment deadlines can create major hassles. First and foremost, you don't want to be without coverage. If you sign up during the OEP or GEP, your coverage won't kick in right away. That can leave you without coverage while you wait for Medicare to go into effect.

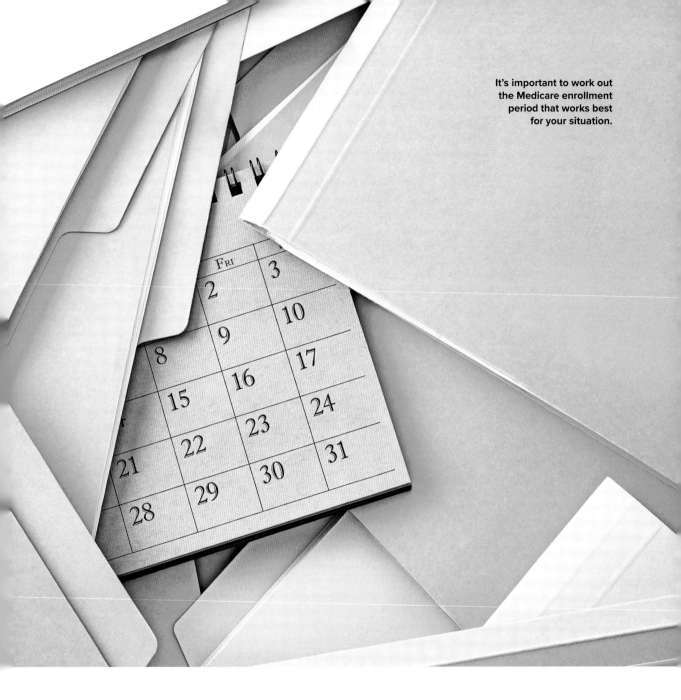

It's important to work out the Medicare enrollment period that works best for your situation.

The second reason to enroll on time is that your premiums will go up the longer that you wait. If you don't enroll during an IEP or SEP, your Part B premium will increase by 10 percentage points for every full 12-month period between the end of your IEP and the end of the GEP during which you finally enrolled. So, for example, if you sign up four years after the end of your IEP, you'll pay 40 percent more in premiums for as long as you are eligible to have Medicare. The only exception to this is if you became eligible before you were 65 due to a disability, in which case the late penalty goes away once you turn 65. ∎

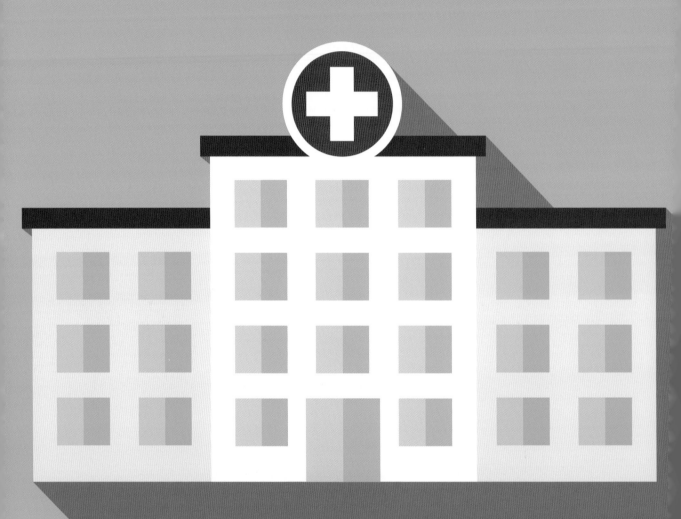

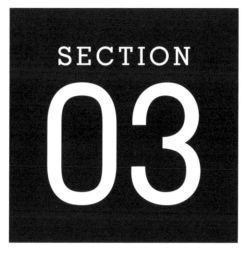

SECTION

03

What Medicare Covers

Understand the different types of plans
and the services they pay for

03 | **MEDICARE PARTS A & B**   01 | 02 | 03 | 04 | 05 | 06

PARTS A & B: AN OVERVIEW Your guide to understanding "Original Medicare"

When people refer to "Original Medicare," they are specifically talking about Medicare Parts A and B. These were the first types of coverage offered when the government program began. Over time, the program has grown to include other coverage options, but Parts A and B still constitute the core of the program. It's worth getting to know them as well as possible.

PART A
What It Covers and What It Costs
Part A is often referred to as "hospital insurance." However, you don't necessarily have to be admitted to a hospital for Part A to cover the services you receive. While Part A covers inpatient care delivered within a hospital, skilled nursing facility or mental health hospital, it also covers home health services and hospice care. Part A covers hospital-related costs as well, including meals provided by the facility, a semi-private room and services such as medical supplies, rehabilitation therapy, lab tests and medical appliances. If the facility itself provides you with prescription drugs, those are also covered under Part A.

Although most people pay no premium for Part A, it is not free care. When you use Part A, you'll have to meet a deductible of $1,408 per period before Medicare begins to cover your care.

Medicare defines a "benefit period" as beginning on the day you're admitted to a hospital or nursing facility on an inpatient basis and ending when you haven't received inpatient care for 60 days in a row. Once a benefit period has ended, if you're newly admitted to a hospital or nursing facility, a new benefit period begins. There's no limit on the number of benefit periods you can have over your lifetime.

Coinsurance payments are extra charges on top of your deductible for Part A. You'll pay them for extended stays in a hospital or skilled nursing facility.

Part A includes additional coinsurance charges after you've paid your deductible. These charges are based on the number of days you receive care during a benefit period. Hospital coinsurance charges are:

- **Days 1–60** $0

- **Days 61–90** $352 per day

- **Days 91 and Beyond** These

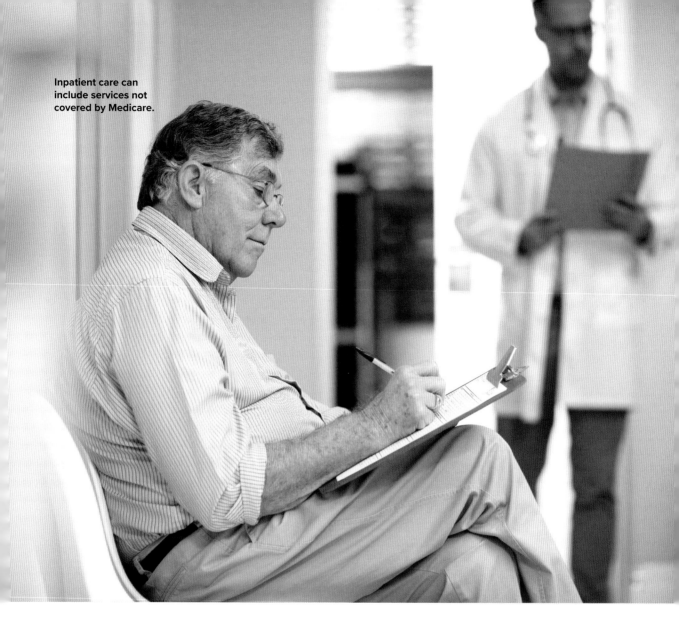

Inpatient care can include services not covered by Medicare.

are called "lifetime reserve days," and they cost $704 each. You only get to use 60 of these during your lifetime.

After you use up your 60 "lifetime reserve days" [see details, above] you pay all costs for inpatient stays that are longer than 90 days in a given benefit period.

Daily coinsurance for care in a skilled nursing facility per benefit period is:

- **Days 1–20** $0

- **Days 21–100** $176

- **Days 101 and Beyond** You pay all costs

For eligible home health services and hospice care, there is no daily coinsurance rate. However, you will pay 5 percent of the Medicare-approved rate for inpatient respite care you receive through hospice.

49

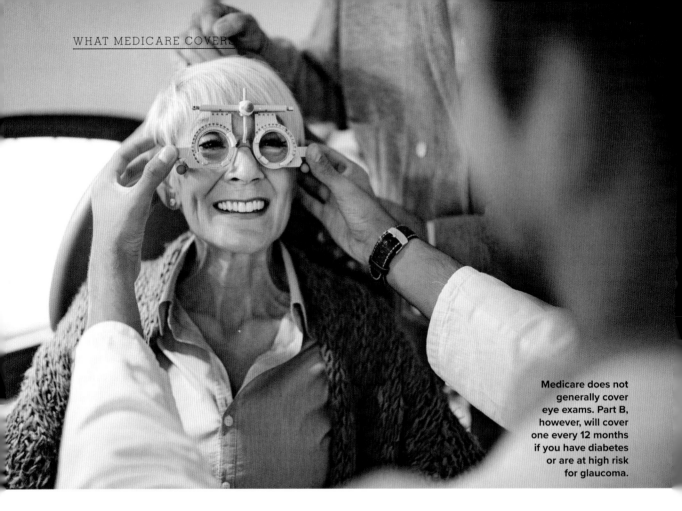

Medicare does not generally cover eye exams. Part B, however, will cover one every 12 months if you have diabetes or are at high risk for glaucoma.

In any inpatient care situation, it is always possible that your doctor will recommend care that Medicare does not cover. Make sure to ask your provider if a specific treatment or service is going to be covered or not, so that you know up-front how much it will cost.

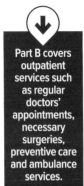

Part B covers outpatient services such as regular doctors' appointments, necessary surgeries, preventive care and ambulance services.

PART B
Coverage and Costs

Part B is the type of coverage you'll likely rely on most while on Medicare. It covers outpatient services, such as doctors' appointments, necessary surgeries, preventive care, outpatient mental-health care and ambulance services. Everyone pays a monthly premium for Part B. For 2020, the standard monthly premium is $144.60. Single individuals earning more than $87,000 per year and married couples making over $174,000 jointly per year will pay more.

On top of your monthly premium, you'll also pay a deductible and a coinsurance fee for any services you receive. Beginning in 2020, the annual deductible for Part B is $198, meaning you'll have to pay $198 out of pocket each year before Medicare begins to cover your care. After you have reached your deductible, the coinsurance rate is 20 percent of the Medicare-approved cost for any service. So, if you've already hit your deductible and require a procedure with a Medicare-approved cost of $200, you'll pay $40 and Medicare will cover the rest.

MEDIGAP

If you've got regular health-care expenses that aren't covered by Medicare Parts A and B, consider a supplemental plan.

Many seniors live on a fixed income—which is why Medicare is meant to be affordable. However, even with its low costs, Medicare's deductibles and coinsurance rates can still be a financial burden. That's why there's also Medigap, also known as Medicare Supplement Insurance. Medigap policies are sold by private insurers, but are strictly regulated by the government. They come in a variety of standardized plans and are built to help cover costs associated with Parts A and B.

Medigap plans are named by letter of the alphabet (much like the different parts of Medicare). They each have a different monthly premium, which reflects their differing levels of benefits. Depending on which plan you sign up for, your Medigap insurance may cover your deductible for Parts A or B, as well as the coinsurance for any services you receive. Medigap plans can also cover things that Original Medicare doesn't cover. For example, while Medicare will cover the cost of getting a blood transfusion, it won't cover the cost of the first 3 pints of blood you receive. Blood is often free, but in the event that you are charged for it, a Medigap plan will cover the first 3 pints.

Medigap plans may offer big savings on health-care costs, but you'll need to sign up within six months of enrolling in Part B. After that, government restrictions no longer apply and you can be denied coverage or charged a higher rate due to your age or a preexisting condition. Whenever you apply, be sure to ask multiple companies for quotes. Just because the plans are standardized doesn't mean the premiums are. Each company calculates its premium costs differently, so it pays to shop around.

What's Not Covered

Before you check into a hospital or other facility, make sure that it accepts Medicare. Otherwise, there's no guarantee you'll be covered. It's also important to note that though Part A does cover care within skilled nursing facilities, this is only true for short-term care. Your Medicare coverage does not extend to long-term care.

Many people are also surprised to learn that Medicare does not cover hearing aids, eye exams, glasses, dental care (including dentures) or routine foot care. For this reason, many Medicare beneficiaries choose to enroll in Medicare Advantage plans that also cover these services. You'll need to choose these plans carefully, however, since not all Medicare Advantage plans cover all services. For prescription drug coverage, you'll also have to enroll in Part D.

If you're worried about being able to cover your deductible or coinsurance for services covered by Parts A and B, you may want to enroll in a Medigap plan, which will help cover those costs. ∎

THE ABCS OF MEDICARE PART D
With the high cost of prescription drugs, many seniors can't afford to be without it

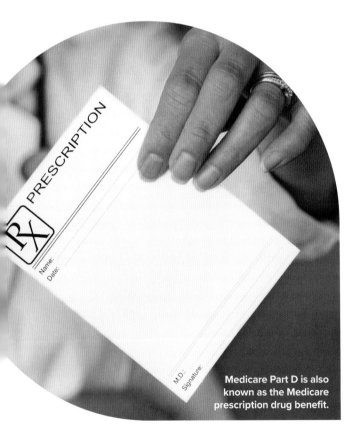

Medicare Part D is also known as the Medicare prescription drug benefit.

Medicare Part D went into effect in 2006 as part of an effort to ensure that beneficiaries wouldn't go broke due to the high cost of prescription drugs. While Part D can help you save you a lot of money on medication, understanding it can also be a bit of a headache. Since Part D is provided by private insurers, the plans vary quite a bit. When selecting a Part D plan, make sure you understand exactly how your plan works, what it covers and how much you can expect to pay for the medicines that you need.

PART D
What It Covers
To be covered by Part D, a medication must be:

• **Prescribed by a Doctor** Part D doesn't cover over-the-counter medications or vitamins.

• **Medically Necessary** Part D does not cover drugs taken for cosmetic reasons or for things like impotence or weight loss.

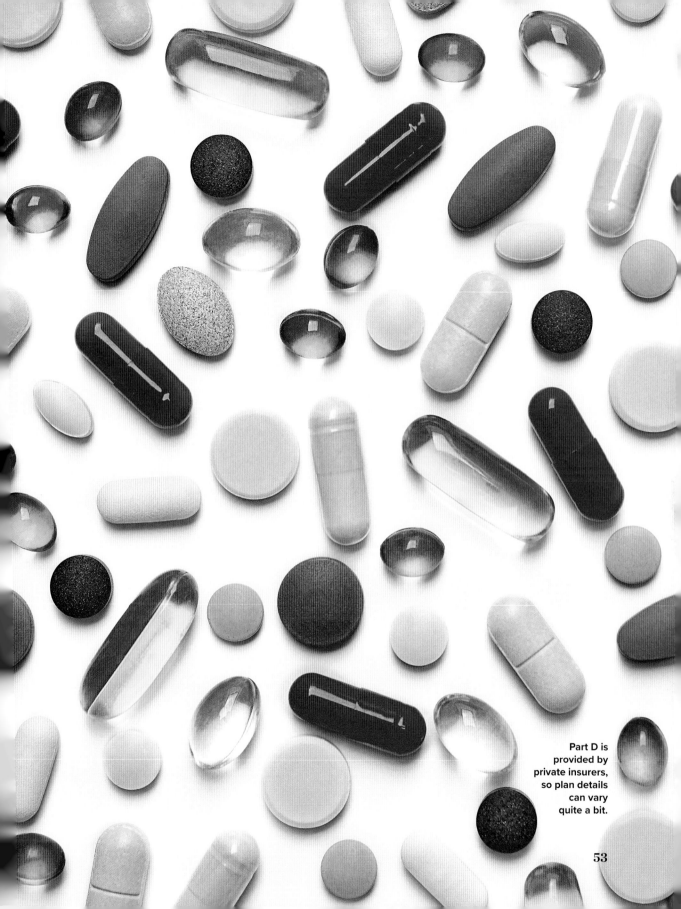

Part D is
provided by
private insurers,
so plan details
can vary
quite a bit.

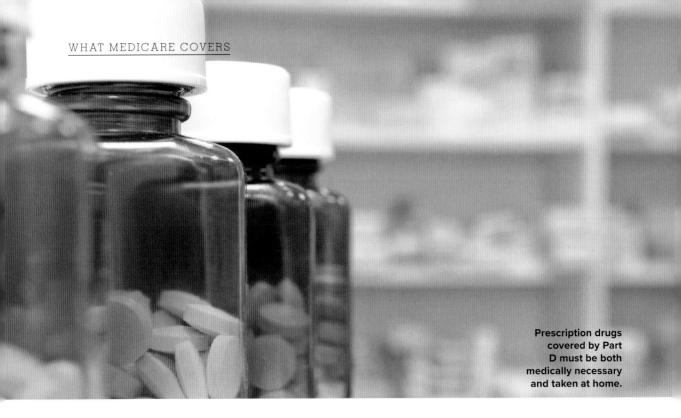

Prescription drugs covered by Part D must be both medically necessary and taken at home.

• **Taken on an Outpatient Basis** Drugs that are administered to you in a hospital or nursing facility are covered under Part A. If you go to a doctor's office for injections of chemotherapy or other medications, those are covered under Part B. Part D only covers drugs that you take at home—such as insulin, antidepressants or other commonly prescribed medications.

Plans aren't required to cover all drugs, but they are required to cover a number of drugs from within each of the following classes:

• HIV/AIDS drugs
• Immunosuppressants
• Anti-cancer drugs
• Anti-convulsants
• Antidepressants
• Antipsychotics

Plans cover both generic and brand-name drugs, and vary in terms of how much they charge for each. The list of drugs that your plan covers is called your plan's formulary. If your doctor de-termines that you need a drug outside of your plan's formulary, you may request an exception from your insurer. When you make the request, you'll have to include a statement describing why the drug is necessary for you to take, and why a similar medication within your plan's formulary isn't suitable for you.

Plans may make changes to their formularies during the year—removing some drugs or adding new ones. If your prescriptions are affected by the changes, you may end up paying more for a medication you've been taking, or you may need to request an exception if your medication is no longer covered.

How to Get Part D

Part D plans are provided by private insurance companies, and plans are strictly regulated by the government to meet certain standards (al-though plans can vary widely from company to company). Most people will sign up for Part D when they sign up for Part B, but if you contin-

THE DONUT HOLE

The coverage gap—also known as the "donut hole"—is a period of time during which your Part D coverage isn't in full effect. Here's how the situation arises.

Once you've paid your yearly deductible, your Part D plan kicks in and helps pay for your medications—but only until the total cost for your prescriptions hits $4,020. That number includes all money spent on your prescriptions—by both you and your insurer. The space between $4,020 and $6,350 in prescription drug costs is the donut hole. It's the space where your plan isn't in full effect yet and your drug costs can still rise: When you're in the donut hole, your plan doesn't provide any coverage. However, you'll still get discounts from the government and drug makers. Once you reach the $5,100 cap on out-of-pocket expenses, coverage kicks back in.

Luckily, Congress has worked to mitigate the effects of the gap, and many consider the donut hole effectively closed as of 2020. That's because people who find themselves in the donut hole will only pay 25 percent of the costs for their drugs, which is the same percentage they pay in coinsurance *before* they hit the coverage gap. (Previously, they would pay 37 percent of the costs of generics and 25 percent for brand names while in the donut hole). What's more, while you're in the donut hole, you will be able to count almost the full price of any brand-name drugs toward your out-of-pocket costs despite receiving a 75-percent discount. That helps get you out of the donut hole as quickly as possible.

After you hit $6,350 in expenses and exit the donut hole, you'll be getting "catastrophic coverage." Your costs for medication will be 5 percent of the drug's cost, or a copay of $3.60 for generics or $8.95 for brand-name drugs—whichever is greater.

ue to have "creditable prescription drug coverage"—meaning drug coverage that is at least as good as Medicare's—through another source, you can delay enrolling in Part D without a late penalty. To help you find a plan, the government offers an online tool, the Medicare Plan Finder (medicare.gov/find-a-plan), which can help you find the plans available where you live.

If you want to drop or change your plan, you can generally only do so during the open enrollment period each year (Oct. 15 to Dec. 7). Some circumstances do allow for changes outside of this time frame—such as if you move outside of your plan's geographical area.

Understanding Costs

Most Part D plans have a monthly premium and a yearly deductible. In 2020, base beneficiary monthly premium for Part D plans is roughly $33. High-income individuals also have to pay the additional Income-Related Monthly Adjustment Amount (IRMAA), required by the government, on top of their premium. Deductibles can vary by plan, but are capped for 2020 at $435.

Part D plans generally separate drugs into different tiers, based on price. In most cases, you'll have a lower copay for generic drugs. Brand-name and more expensive drugs will often come with higher copays or coinsurance rates. ∎

WHAT MEDICARE DOESN'T COVER
The program covers many health expenses— with some important exceptions

Medicare covers a large portion of your medical costs after you turn 65, but the program doesn't cover everything. Understanding the scope and limits of your Medicare coverage can help you plan for additional costs.

One important distinction you should understand: If custodial care—help with daily activities, such as dressing, bathing, cooking and laundry—is the only care you need, Medicare does not cover it. Most nursing home care is considered custodial care.

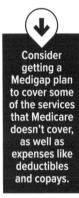

Consider getting a Medigap plan to cover some of the services that Medicare doesn't cover, as well as expenses like deductibles and copays.

However, Medicare does cover skilled nursing services, defined as medically necessary care ordered by a doctor and conducted under the supervision of a medical professional, such as a nurse or physical therapist. In fact, Medicare covers up to 100 days of care in a skilled nursing facility each benefit period, as long as you were admitted to the hospital

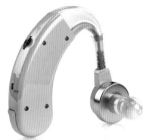

Many Medicare Advantage plans offer at least basic hearing, vision and dental benefits.

for at least three days first. Likewise, Medicare Parts A and B don't cover the following: :

- Dental care, including dentures
- Routine vision
- Hearing aids
- Long-term care
- Foreign travel emergencies
- Cosmetic surgery
- Most chiropractic services
- Acupuncture
- Routine foot care

Many Medicare Advantage plans offer some, but not extensive, vision and dental benefits. A supplemental Medigap policy can help fill the gaps where Medicare leaves off, providing coverage for out-of-pocket expenses such as copays, deductibles and coinsurance. ∎

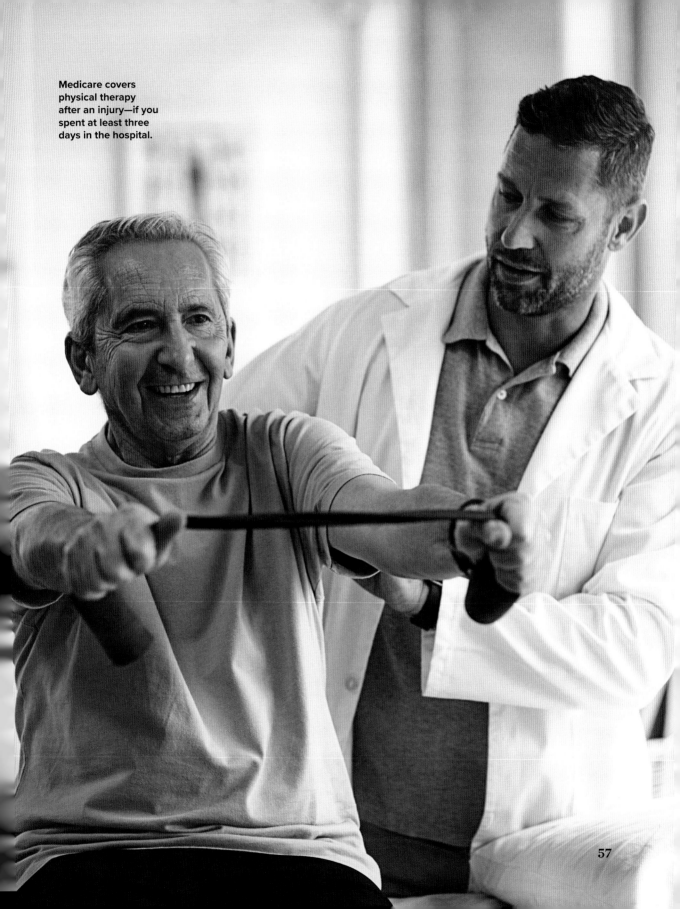

Medicare covers physical therapy after an injury—if you spent at least three days in the hospital.

03 | MEDICARE ADVANTAGE 01 | 02 | 03 | 04 | 05 | 06

PART C: MEDICARE ADVANTAGE
What additional coverage you can (and can't) expect from these plans

Original Medicare doesn't cover some common health-care needs, such as dental care, vision care and hearing aids. To get coverage for these items, you may want to consider a Medicare Advantage (MA) plan, also known as Part C. MA plans are run by private insurers, and by law they must provide at least the same benefits and protections as Original Medicare. Most MA plans attract participants by covering additional services as well, including prescription drugs, which would normally be covered by Part D.

To join an MA plan, you must be enrolled in Original Medicare. You can use the Medicare website's Plan Finder by visiting medicare.gov/find-a-plan to locate and research plans available in your area. Once you join one, you'll still pay your Part B premium, but you'll pay a separate monthly premium for your MA plan, if it charges

Use the Medicare website's Plan Finder to locate and research Medicare Advantage plans that are offered in your geographical area.

one (some do and some don't). If at any point you want to change plans or go back to Original Medicare, you can do so from Jan. 1 to March 31 each year. And remember, you're still considered "on Medicare" even if you have an MA plan.

There are five main types of MA plans. Each operates in its own way and you'll need to decide which style is best for you. Here are the common types of plans among which most people enrolling in MA can choose:

• **Health Maintenance Organizations (HMOs)** These plans require you to use doctors and other providers within their network, except in the case of an emergency. They may also require a referral before you can go to certain specialists.

• **Preferred Provider Organizations (PPOs)** In these plans, you'll pay less when you use a provider within the plan's network and more when you use one outside the network.

• **Private Fee-For-Service (PFFS)** Much like original Medicare, these plans let you choose

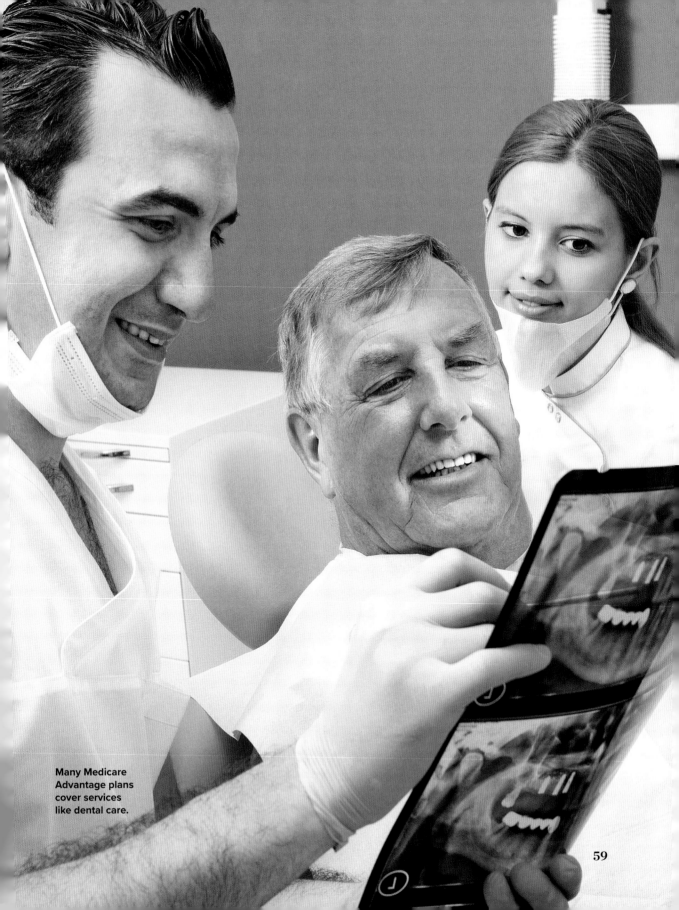

Many Medicare Advantage plans cover services like dental care.

59

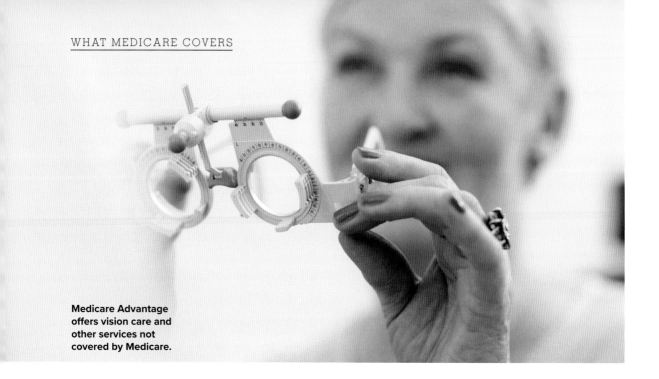

Medicare Advantage offers vision care and other services not covered by Medicare.

where you'll receive care (as long as the health-care provider accepts your plan). The plan sets the rates it will pay for each service, as well as any costs you'll have to bear, such as copayments.

• **Special Needs Plans (SNPs)** These plans are less common and are for people with specific circumstances—such as those living in nursing homes or receiving Medicaid.

• **Medical Savings Accounts (MSAs)** These plans give you a bank account into which they deposit funds that you may use to cover your health-care costs. They generally have a high deductible, so you'll likely use everything in the bank account (and then some) before your coverage kicks in. But once you reach your deductible, the plan covers 100 percent of your costs.

Medicare Disadvantage?

Even though all MA plans cover everything included in Original Medicare, they're still free to create their own restrictions or charge higher coinsurance rates than Original Medicare. Depending on your health, your out-of-pocket costs may increase. Luckily, the government limits how much an MA plan can allow you to spend. For example, in 2020, the maximum out-of-pocket cost for a person with an HMO plan is $6,700.

Many MA plans have no monthly premium, which can seem appealing at first. However, people enrolled in these plans often see their costs shoot up once they get sick, because the plans often compensate with high coinsurance or copay rates for some services. This type of fee structure can translate to low costs while you're healthy but end up generating much higher costs as soon as you need care.

Another disadvantage of MA plans can be finding care while away from home. Many retirees travel or enjoy being "snowbirds," but most MA plans are limited to specific geographical areas—meaning you may need to fly home for care if you get sick during your fun in the sun.

Finally, keep in mind that Medigap and MA plans are mutually exclusive—it's illegal for someone to sell you one if you have the other. So research all of your options before you enroll. ∎

MEDIGAP COVERAGE Supplemental insurance to reduce your out-of-pocket costs

Also known as Medicare supplemental insurance, Medigap policies can help you save money on out-of-pocket expenses. Private insurers offer these plans as a way for seniors to help fill in the gaps of their Medicare coverage. When you select one, you remain enrolled in Parts A and B (and still pay your Part B premium). But you'll also pay a premium to your Medigap provider, which entitles you to extra benefits. It's also important to note that plans sold after 2006 can't cover prescription drugs, so you'll also need to enroll in Part D to achieve complete coverage.

> As with other types of insurance, plans with fewer benefits have lower premiums, and plans with more benefits have higher premiums.

Some Medigap plans cover expenses not covered by Original Medicare (such as coverage for emergency care overseas). All plans help cover costs related to parts A and B (such as coinsurance and copayments). Because these plans have the potential to cover many out-of-pocket costs, insurance companies are strict about when you can enroll.

The government prohibits insurers from denying coverage (or raising premiums based on health or age) for the first six months after you've enrolled in Part B. Because of this policy, to be eligible for any Medigap policy in your area, you must sign up within six months of enrolling in Part B. After that date, insurers can refuse to offer you a plan.

Types of Plans

All Medigap plans are standardized—each must offer a specific set of benefits regulated by the government. However, costs can vary by company, and depending on where you live. Companies price their policies in different ways as well, so explore all of your options before choosing one.

There are 10 different types of plans and they're identified by letters of the alphabet, ranging from A to N. Plan A offers the fewest benefits, while Plan F currently offers the most. As with other types of insurance, your benefits will generally reflect how much of a premium you pay: Plans with fewer benefits have lower premiums, while plans with more benefits have higher premiums.

Medigap plans can cover most or all of the out-of-pocket costs that Original Medicare doesn't

Medigap plans can help cover out-of-pocket costs Original Medicare won't pay for.

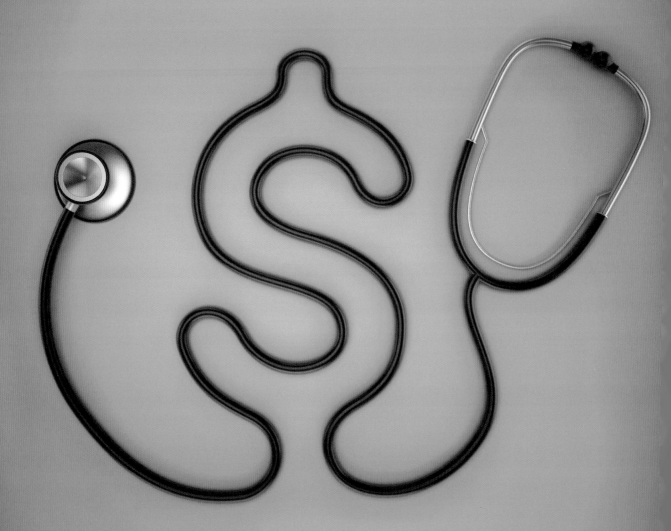

All Medigap plans are standardized—each must offer a specific set of benefits.

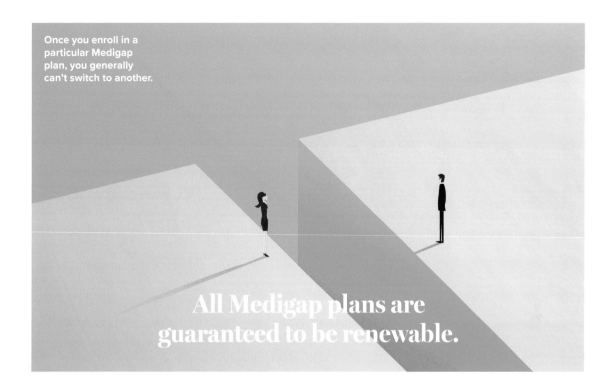

Once you enroll in a particular Medigap plan, you generally can't switch to another.

All Medigap plans are guaranteed to be renewable.

cover. For example, some plans cover the entire cost of your Part A and/or Part B deductible, as well as your copayments and coinsurance. With the right plan (and depending on your health), your out-of-pocket expenses could approach zero some years—aside from your premiums.

Note that Wisconsin, Massachusetts and Minnesota standardize Medigap differently than the rest of the country, so plans available in those states will have different standards of care and will go by different names.

Changing Plans

Generally, once you're enrolled in a Medigap plan, you can't switch to another. You may qualify for an exception to this rule if you're still within your six-month enrollment period or have "guaranteed issue rights" due to other circumstances. You may have guaranteed issue rights if your Medigap insurance company goes bankrupt, or if you've been on a Medicare Advantage plan but have moved out of the plan's service area.

However, if you no longer wish to be enrolled in Medigap, you can drop your plan and opt to sign up for a Medicare Advantage plan during open enrollment instead.

Medigap plans are guaranteed renewable, meaning your insurer can't drop you or discontinue your policy unless you stop paying your premium or were fraudulent in your application. Occasionally, the government makes changes to the benefits offered by Medigap plans, or even discontinues an existing plan offering entirely. Generally, if you are enrolled in a plan that gets discontinued by the government, you'll be grandfathered in, meaning you will be able to stay in that plan without having to make any changes. You won't be able to change to any discontinued plan, nor will it accept any new enrollees. ■

MEDICARE VS. MEDICAID One is for seniors, the other is for low-income Americans

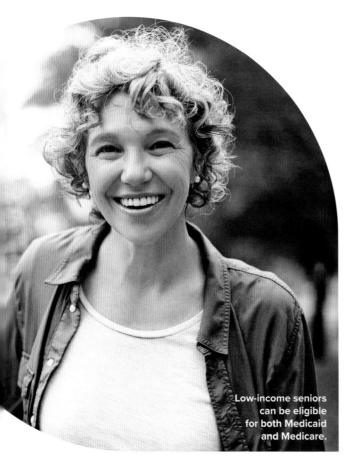

Low-income seniors can be eligible for both Medicaid and Medicare.

Medicare and Medicaid sound alike and have some similarities, but they are two different programs. Both are government-funded and designed to help cover health-care costs for American citizens, but they differ in exactly how they are funded and in whom they serve.

Medicare is funded by the federal government and offers health-care coverage to those 65 and older. Medicaid is a joint federal and state program that provides care for low-income Americans, children, pregnant women and people with disabilities. Because Medicaid is jointly funded by the federal government and states, each state operates its own program and eligibility requirements vary. While Medicare is available to nearly every American age 65 and older regardless of income level, Medicaid is based primarily on financial need, so recipients must meet their state's income-eligibility requirements to qualify. In many states, recipients cannot have more than a few thousand dollars in liquid assets in order to participate in Medicaid.

Medicaid typically covers medical services at no cost to the recipient, though in some states a

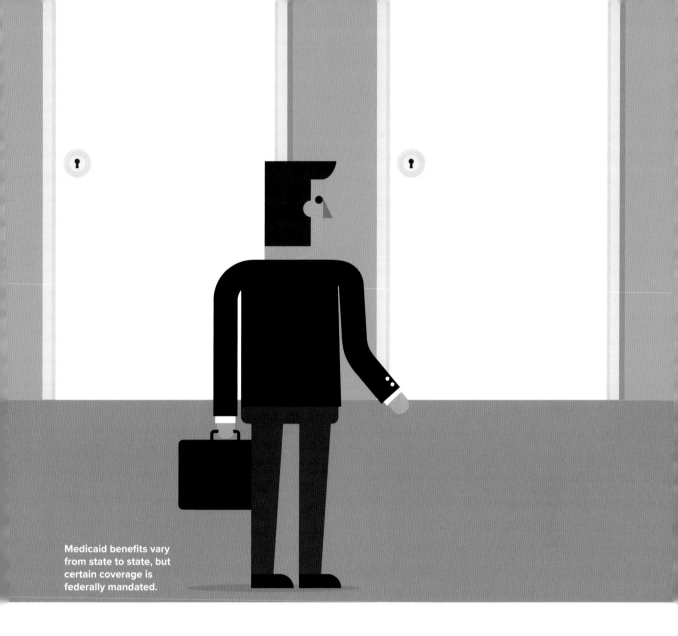

Medicaid benefits vary from state to state, but certain coverage is federally mandated.

small copayment may be required. Medicaid benefits vary by state, but the federal government mandates coverage of hospitalizations; doctor services; nursing services; laboratory services; family planning; X-rays; pediatric and family nurse practitioner services; and clinic treatment. Medicaid also offers coverage for two types of care Medicare does not: custodial care and nursing home care. States can also choose to provide additional services beyond the mandatory requirements set by the federal government, such as prescription drug coverage, dental care, or physical and occupational therapy.

Low-income seniors can be eligible for both Medicaid and Medicare; in that case, Medicaid will help cover some of the costs associated with Medicare. If you need assistance with Medicare-related costs but don't qualify for Medicaid, you may qualify for your state's Medicare Savings Program. To learn more about Medicare Savings Programs, contact your state Medicaid office. ∎

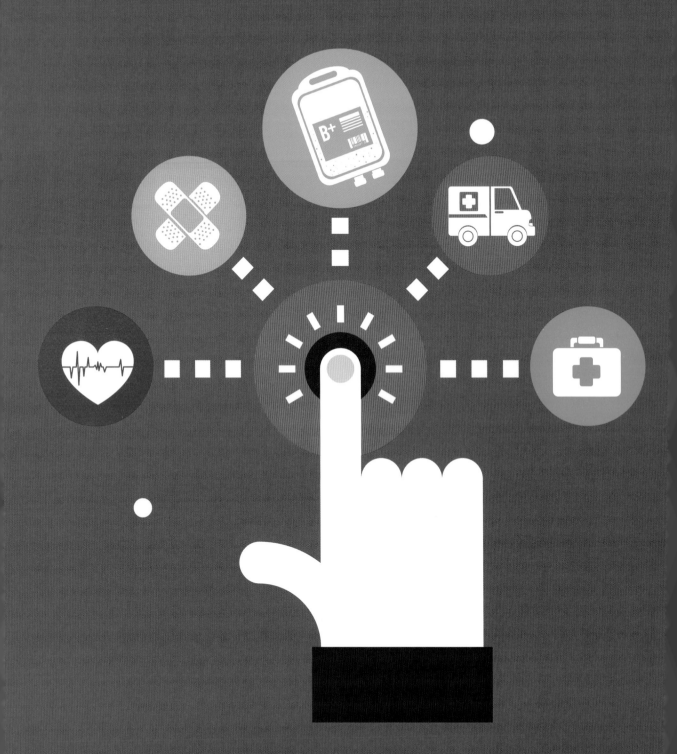

Choosing the Right Coverage

How to pick a Medicare plan, or a combination of plans, to meet your needs

04 | **PLAN OVERVIEWS** | 01 | 02 | 03 | 04 | 05 | 06

PICKING YOUR PLANS How to combine the different types of Medicare

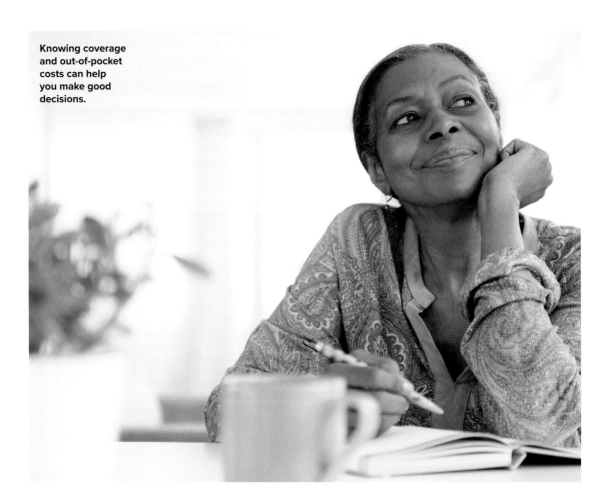

Knowing coverage and out-of-pocket costs can help you make good decisions.

If You Have...	What's Covered	Out-of-Pocket Costs (including premiums)	Pros	Cons
PART A & B ONLY (ORIGINAL MEDICARE)	• Inpatient care in hospitals, skilled nursing facilities, home health services • Outpatient care	• Deductible of $1,408 per benefit period for Part A and $198 per year for Part B	• Care is covered anywhere in the country • No need for referrals to see a specialist	• Some health-care needs, such as prescription drugs, aren't covered • Limitless out-of-pocket expenses
PART A, B & D	• Everything above, plus outpatient prescription drugs	• Deductible of $1,408 per benefit period for Part A and $198 per year for Part B • Deductibles/copays for RXs vary by plan	• Same as above	• Limitless out-of-pocket expenses
PART A, B, D & MEDIGAP	• Everything above, plus some out-of-pocket costs, such as coinsurance and deductibles • Coverage varies by plan	• Some Medigap plans cover your deductibles; all provide some coinsurance coverage	• Same as above • Medigap plans that cover deductibles can mean some care is completely free	• No limit on out-of-pocket expenses • Changing Medigap plans can be hard after six months
PART C (MEDICARE ADVANTAGE)	• All plans must cover everything that Parts A and B cover. Most include Part D • Some plans also cover vision, dental and hearing services	• Up to $6,700	• Out-of-pocket expenses are limited to $6,700 per year • Ability to switch between plans each year during open enrollment	• Covered care limited to in-network providers • Networks only cover certain geographical areas • Specialists require referrals

UNDERSTANDING THE COSTS Know what to expect when your health care bill arrives

How much Medicare costs depends on how you structure your coverage. While you can't fully anticipate the care you'll need down the road, you can balance the potential costs with the best possible coverage option.

PART A
Premium-Free, but Not Cost-Free

Most people won't pay any monthly premium for Part A because they or a spouse have paid Medicare payroll taxes while they were working. However, if you or your spouse haven't earned premium-free Part A, you'll typically have to pay the following monthly premiums:

• **$458** if you worked fewer than 30 quarters

• **$252** if you worked between 30 and 39 quarters

Everyone pays a deductible for Part A, regardless of whether or not they pay a premium. The deductible per benefit period is $1,408. In other words, you'll pay $1,408 out of pocket before Medicare starts chipping in. Once you've met this deductible, Part A covers inpatient costs.

You'll also pay coinsurance based on how many days you've been in the hospital during that benefit period:

• **Days 1–60** $0

• **Days 61–90** $352 per day

• **Days 91 and Beyond** Called "lifetime reserve days," they cost $704 each. You only get to use 60 of these during your lifetime.

• **Beyond Reserve** When your 60 lifetime reserve days are gone, you pay all costs for inpatient stays longer than 90 days in a given benefit period.

Daily coinsurance for care in a skilled nursing facility per benefit period is:

• **Days 1–20** $0

• **Days 21–100** $176

• **Days 101 and Beyond** You pay all costs.

There is no daily coinsurance rate for home health services or hospice.

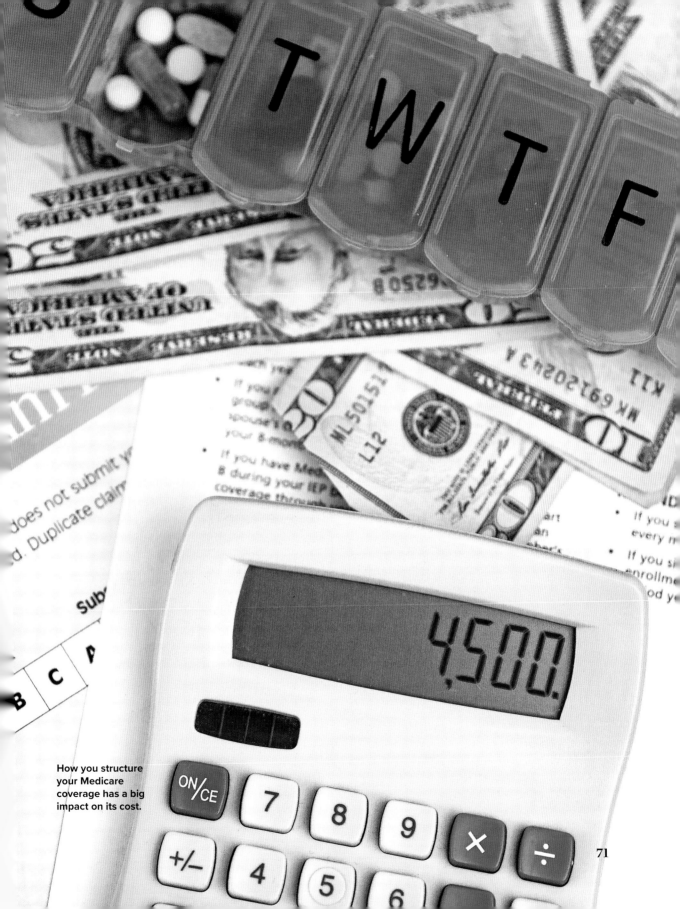

How you structure your Medicare coverage has a big impact on its cost.

71

PART B

Outpatient Care

Everyone has to pay a monthly premium for Part B. The cost of these premiums usually goes up a little bit each year to account for inflation. In 2020, the standard monthly premium is $144.60. However, those making more than $87,000 per year (or $174,000 as a couple filing jointly) will pay more. Medicare refers to this higher rate as the Medicare Income-Related Monthly Adjustment Amount (IRMAA). It applies for both Parts B and D, and Medicare will alert you if you need to pay it. For monthly Part B premiums adjusted for IRMAA, see the table on opposite page.

In addition to your monthly premiums, you'll also have a deductible, coinsurance and copayments. Unlike with Part A, you don't need to worry about "benefit periods," since Part B's costs are calculated annually. For example, all Medicare subscribers' deductible for Part B is $198, which means you'll have to pay $198 out-of-pocket each year before Medicare begins to pay the bills. After you've met your deductible, Part B will pay 80 percent of most of your outpatient health care costs and you'll pay 20 percent.

However, there are exceptions:

• **Preventive Care** Many services recommended by the U.S. Preventive Services Task Force are covered 100 percent by Medicare.

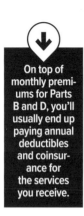

On top of monthly premiums for Parts B and D, you'll usually end up paying annual deductibles and coinsurance for the services you receive.

• **Outpatient Hospital Care** You'll pay coinsurance up to $1,408 (the same as your Part A deductible) if you seek outpatient care at a hospital.

• **Qualifying Home Health Services** If covered by Part B, these services are 100 percent covered and can include physical therapy, occupational therapy and part-time home health aide services.

• **Care Provided by a Non-Participating Provider** Some providers accept Medicare but do not "take assignment." That means they may charge up to 15 percent more than the Medicare-approved amount for a service. In this situation, you'll pay 35 percent of the cost of your care (the usual 20 percent, plus 15 percent of the Medicare-approved cost) and Medicare will cover the rest.

Before agreeing to a procedure or appointment, always check with your provider to make certain you understand what is and isn't covered.

PART D

Paying for Prescriptions

Because Part D plans are sold by private insurers, they have different monthly premiums. In 2020, the base beneficiary premium for a Part D plan is around $33.

As with Part B, individuals with incomes over $87,000 per year (or $174,000 jointly) will have to also pay the IRMAA required by the government. The amount of your IRMAA depends on your income. (See the table on page 74 for the IRMAA amounts for 2020.)

Plans also generally have an annual deductible, which for 2020 may not exceed $435. Some Part D plans don't have a deductible, in which case you won't pay anything out of pocket before your coverage begins. Once you've met any deductible you need to pay, you'll also pay coinsurance or copays as determined by your insurer.

Part D plans can vary in how they structure cost-sharing. However, every plan must meet or exceed the standard of benefits set by the federal government. A standard plan will have a $435 deductible and you'll pay a coinsurance rate of 25 percent (while they cover the rest). Nonstandard plans can use other types of cost-sharing structures, but the federal government must judge that their benefits are "actuarially equivalent" to standard plans.

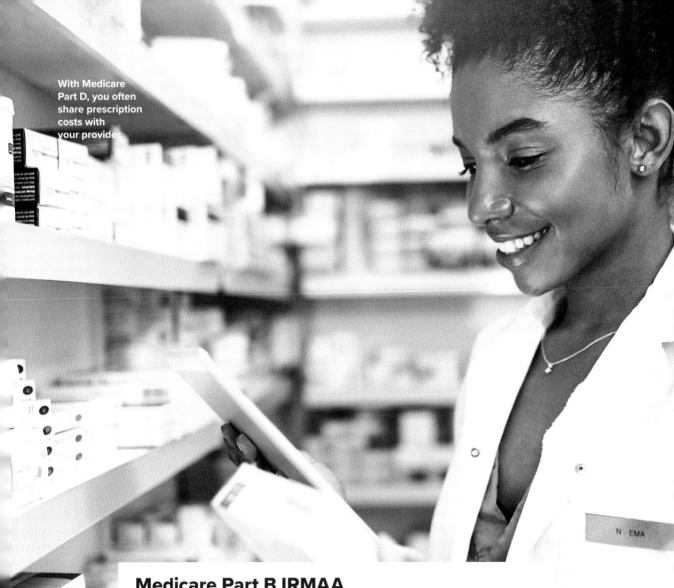

With Medicare Part D, you often share prescription costs with your provider.

Medicare Part B IRMAA

Individual Income	Joint Income for Married Couples	Monthly Part B Premium
$87,001 – $109,000	$174,001 – $218,000	$202.40
$109,001 – $136,000	$218,001 – $272,000	$289.20
$136,001 – $163,000	$272,001 – $326,000	$376.00
$163,001 – $499,999	$326,001 – $749,999	$462.70
At or above $500,000	At or above $750,000	$491.60

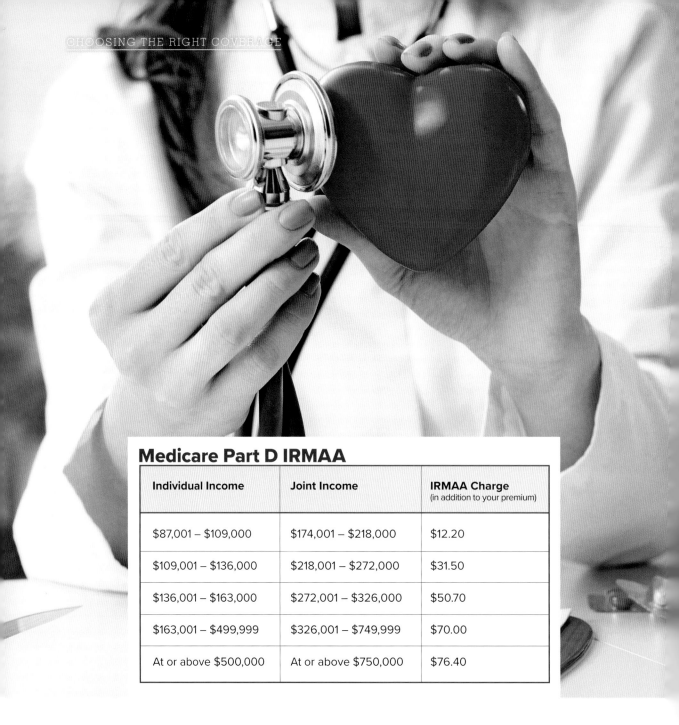

Medicare Part D IRMAA

Individual Income	Joint Income	IRMAA Charge (in addition to your premium)
$87,001 – $109,000	$174,001 – $218,000	$12.20
$109,001 – $136,000	$218,001 – $272,000	$31.50
$136,001 – $163,000	$272,001 – $326,000	$50.70
$163,001 – $499,999	$326,001 – $749,999	$70.00
At or above $500,000	At or above $750,000	$76.40

With any Part D plan, you'll continue to share the costs of your prescriptions until you and your plan have jointly contributed a total of $4,020. At that point, you will fall into the donut hole—but as of 2020, you will only be required to continue to pay no more than 25 percent of costs. Once your total prescription drug costs get to $6,350, you will qualify for catastrophic drug coverage. If that happens, you will pay only 5 percent of the drug's cost, or $3.60 for generic

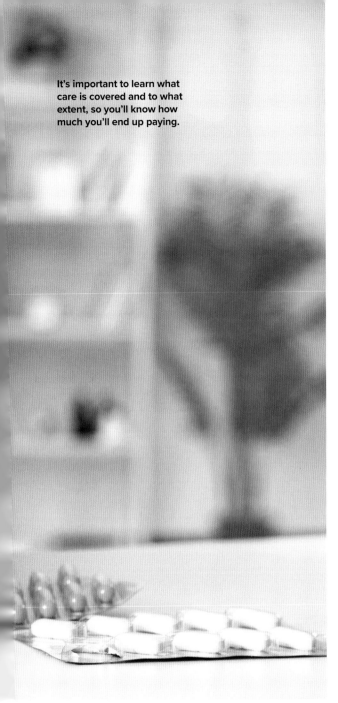

It's important to learn what care is covered and to what extent, so you'll know how much you'll end up paying.

A Sample Cost Calculation

Let's say you have premium-free Part A and have not been admitted to a hospital in the past six months. One day, you have trouble breathing and are admitted to a hospital for five days. After five days, they send you home with a referral to see a cardiologist. The bill you receive for services in the hospital totals $10,500. You'll pay the first $1,408 of the bill (your Part A deductible) and Medicare will cover the rest, since you're within your first 60 days of inpatient care for the benefit period.

Say you then go to an outpatient cardiologist appointment. The doctor performs a $1,200 echocardiogram. Since you haven't had any other outpatient care this year, you'll pay the first $198 of that bill (your Part B deductible), leaving $1,002 remaining. Of this $1,002, you'll pay 20 percent ($200) and Medicare will pay 80 percent ($802).

Your total payment for this appointment is $398. You'll only pay 20 percent of the cost for follow-up appointment next month, because you have already met your annual deductible.

Next, say your doctor prescribes a heart medication, and a three-month prescription for the generic version of the medication costs $140. Your plan doesn't have a deductible and only requires a $10 copay for any generic prescriptions. You'll pay $10.

Your total out-of-pocket expenses, from hospital to prescription costs (not including monthly premiums):

• **$1,408** Hospital stay deductible

• **$398** Cardiologist appointment and echocardiogram

• **$10** Three-month prescription

• **$1,816** Total ∎

drugs, or $8.95 for brand-name drugs—whichever is ultimately considered to be more expensive. And when the year ends, your coverage automatically resets and you will once again need to meet your deductible.

ORIGINAL MEDICARE VS. MEDICARE ADVANTAGE Two options, many possibilities

Deciding which style of Medicare is best for you is a personal choice that depends on a number of factors, including your health, your income and your lifestyle. Consider the following factors when making your selection.

PART C
What's the Advantage?

Medicare Advantage (MA) plans, also known as Medicare Part C, are private insurance plans. To qualify as approved MA plans, they must cover everything included in Original Medicare. Most MA plans cover everything included in a Part D plan as well, and many offer coverage for benefits like vision and dental care, which no part of Original Medicare covers.

Medicare Advantage plans can have surprisingly low premiums. The average monthly premium in 2019 was approximately $29 (plus the standard Part B premium). Couple that with the mandatory limit on out-of-pocket expenses, and an MA plan can promise low costs for comprehensive care. Some plans will even pay for some of your Part B premium.

When you're enrolled in Medicare Advantage, out-of-pocket expenses are limited to $6,700 per year. This amount is known as the maximum out of pocket, or MOOP. Many plans set their own MOOPs well below $6,700. Limiting out-of-pocket costs can save you a significant amount of money—particularly if you need costly surgery or chemotherapy. Original Medicare, on the other hand, has no limit on out-of-pocket costs.

ORIGINAL MEDICARE
No Networks, No Referrals

If Part C has so much to offer, why would anyone still enroll in Original Medicare? There are a few good reasons. First, Original Medicare doesn't limit where you can get care. You can visit any doctor or hospital anywhere in the country as long as they accept Medicare. You won't have to worry about networks or about getting a referral to see a specialist. This flexibility is an important feature for many Medicare users.

Many people also consider Original Medicare to be more stable than Medicare Advantage. MA plans can change their policies and providers can leave MA plans whenever they want. In other words, at any time, you could get a letter explain-

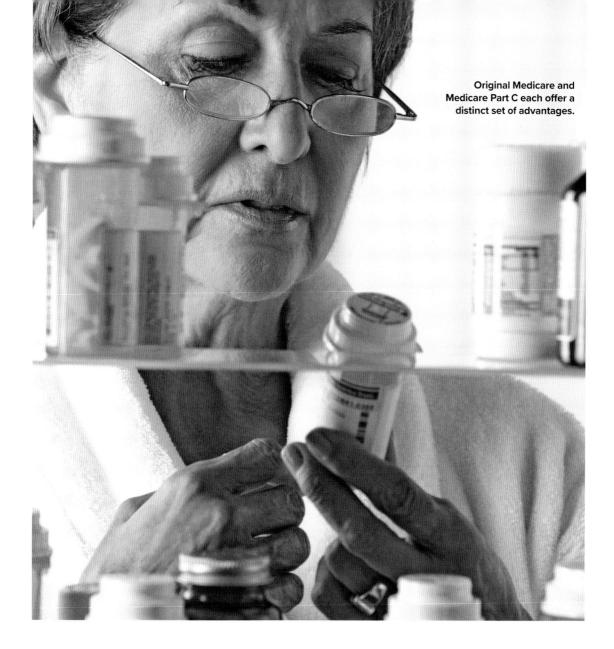

Original Medicare and Medicare Part C each offer a distinct set of advantages.

ing that your preferred doctor is no longer with your plan. You may be granted a special enrollment period to find a new plan, but if you're already dealing with an illness or injury, who needs the extra hassle?

If you want the stability and flexibility of Original Medicare *and* the low cost of an MA plan, a Medigap policy may be the answer. Medigap policies can only be applied to Original Medi-

care (never to Part C) and they can significantly reduce your out-of-pocket costs. For example, a Medigap B Plan covers both your Part A deductible and your coinsurance for hospital stays—making even a lengthy hospital stay free of charge (other than the Medigap plan's premium). If the annual limit on out-of-pocket costs is important to you, Medigap plans K and L offer maximum out-of-pocket costs comparable to those for MAs. ■

04 | **CHOOSING A PART D PLAN** | 01 | 02 | 03 | 04 | 05 | 06

CHOOSING A PART D PLAN
When it comes to prescription drug coverage, the Medicare Plan Finder is your friend

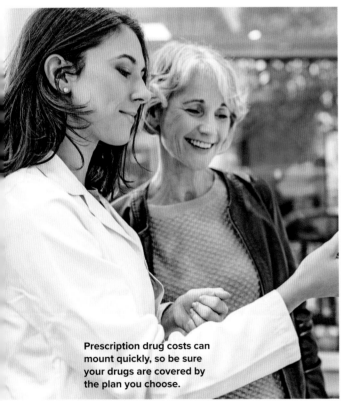

Prescription drug costs can mount quickly, so be sure your drugs are covered by the plan you choose.

When Medicare Part D was created in 2003, many worried there would not be enough plans available to choose from. The concept of prescription drug coverage for Medicare beneficiaries struck both lawmakers and insurance companies as an unprofitable prospect, so the law that created Part D also included a clause that guaranteed at least two plans would be available in every service area—even if the government had to create one.

Since then, the number of Part D plans has exploded, and many people find themselves with more than 20 plans to choose from. With so many options—and all the structural complications of Part D—choosing the most cost-effective plan can be difficult. Luckily, the government provides a useful tool to help you navigate them all: the Medicare Plan Finder (medicare.gov/find-a-plan).

Why the Medicare Plan Finder Is Important
The Medicare Plan Finder is the only online tool that can provide you with a complete, unbiased

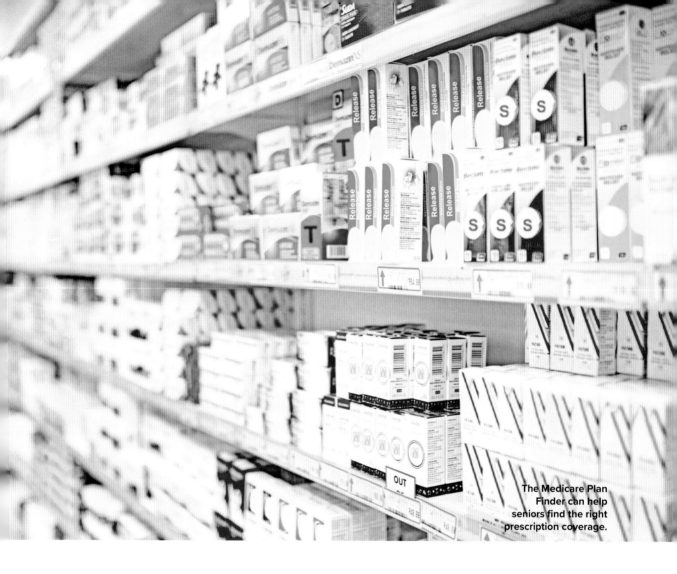

The Medicare Plan Finder can help seniors find the right prescription coverage.

list of all the plans available to you. It's run by the government and is not sponsored by an insurance company, drug company or pharmacy. Everyone who has a stake in Medicare uses the Plan Finder, from beneficiaries to doctors to pharmacies, so Medicare officials continually update the information and monitor it for inaccurate or misleading details. It even includes a star-based rating system that ranks plans based on factors such as accuracy of information and customer satisfaction.

When searching for a Part D plan, many people initially avoid using the Plan Finder because it seems tedious and complicated. Sure, entering all your information—including the dosages and fre-

quency of your medications—isn't anyone's idea of a good time. However, doing so can ultimately save you a lot of cash, and it definitely will save you the headache of calling multiple insurers for quotes.

If you struggle to make sense of online tools, don't despair. Social workers and health care providers have access to the Plan Finder, too. They should be able to help you navigate it to determine which plan is best for you.

Determining the Best Plan
If you're choosing a stand-alone Part D plan (rather than getting Part D through Medicare

Advantage), use the Plan Finder to determine which plans are available to you based on where you live. Generally, the Plan Finder will show you all the plans available in your area and will generally rank them from lowest cost to highest.

But don't stop there! Before you choose the least-expensive option, it's worth taking a closer look. For example, if money is not your top concern and you are more interested in having a top-quality plan, you can ask the Plan Finder to sort according to each plan's star rating. You may find that for only a few dollars more, you can get a plan that ranks well above whatever your least-expensive option is. Additionally, if you see a plan with a gold star icon (meaning that it's earned a coveted five-star rating), you can switch to that plan at any time (except between Dec. 1 and Dec. 7). You don't need to wait for open enrollment, which can be great news if it's early in the year and you're already unhappy with your plan.

You can also see which plans cover drugs nationwide if you use an in-network pharmacy chain. If you travel a lot or spend your winters elsewhere, this benefit could save you money when you need to refill a prescription away from your primary home.

Using the Plan Finder to Understand Your Costs

Part of the Plan Finder's magic lies in its ability to show you how much you'll pay for your medications throughout the year. Since the prices of your drugs change based on how much you've spent in a given year, it's helpful to see the bar graphs that the Plan Finder provides. Each graph is based on the information you entered about your medications. For each plan, it will show you when you'll reach your deductible, when you'll fall into the donut hole, when you'll qualify for catastrophic care, and how much you'll pay out of pocket during each of these phases.

If none of the plans seems affordable to you, there are ways to lower your costs. Once you're looking at the Plan Finder page that details a plan's costs, click the link at the bottom that says "Lower your drug costs." When you click on this link, the Plan Finder will offer you a list of potential resources for lowering your drug costs with that plan, including available generic versions of your medications, patient-assistance programs from drug manufacturers, and local pharmacy assistance programs. Of course, you should consider all the charts shown by the Plan Finder to be estimates—the prices aren't set in stone. And always check with your health care provider about whether a generic or similar drug will work for you before you assume you can switch to the less expensive option.

Knowing Your Preferred Pharmacies

Part D plans generally have "preferred" pharmacies, which will offer a lower copay than other in-network pharmacies. When you initially enter all of your information in the Plan Finder, you'll also have to enter the names of some pharmacies in your area—but you won't know at that point which are in-network for each plan.

When the Plan Finder shows you the details page for a given plan, it'll show you which of your listed pharmacies are preferred, which are in-network, and which aren't covered by that plan. This 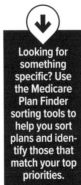 information can have a significant impact on the costs—or convenience—of getting your medications. For example, the closest pharmacy to you may not be in-network for the plan you want. Depending on the distance to the closest preferred pharmacy and the cost of your medications, it may be worth considering whether the cost of a plan that includes your local pharmacy is worth it. You

Looking for something specific? Use the Medicare Plan Finder sorting tools to help you sort plans and identify those that match your top priorities.

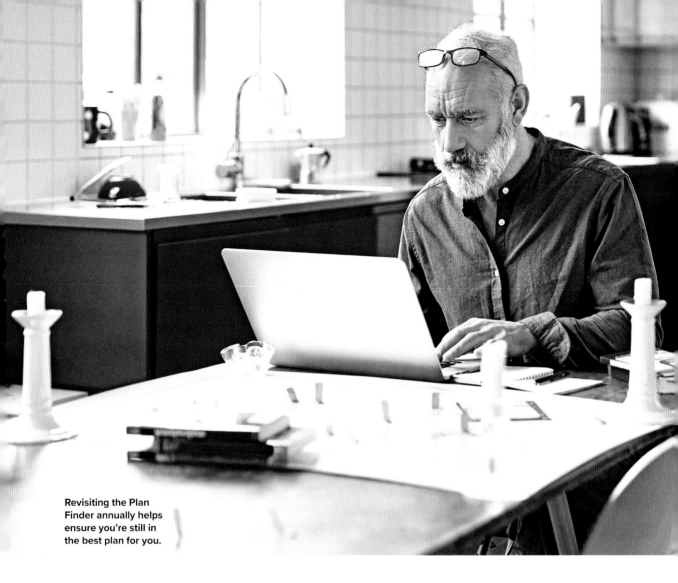

Revisiting the Plan Finder annually helps ensure you're still in the best plan for you.

may want to try filling out the Plan Finder a few times, choosing different pharmacies each time. Remember, your least-expensive plan may change based on which plans prefer which pharmacies.

Staying on Top of Your Options

Over time, Part D plans can change the collection of specific drugs they cover, known as their formulary. Each September, you'll receive a letter from your insurer alerting you to any changes in the plan. You may also get a letter at another point during the year if your plan drops a medication you take. If you don't like your plan, or are unhap-

py with the changes, you can change Part D plans during open enrollment, which begins in October.

Even if you like your plan, it's a good idea to re-enter your information in the Plan Finder each year to make sure you're still enrolled in the best Part D plan for you. Maybe you started taking a new prescription, or another plan has a new mix of benefits that could lower your total costs. Since you're generally only able to switch plans during open enrollment, you may want to mark your calendar to be sure you take stock of your prescription drug coverage options in time to make changes. ∎

SELECTING A MEDIGAP PLAN There are plenty of options for filling the holes

Those sticking with Original Medicare will almost certainly also want to enroll in Medigap. Also known as Medicare Supplement Insurance, Medigap plans were designed to help ease out-of-pocket costs, and sometimes they will even cover deductibles. Medigap plans are standardized by the government, so the benefits will be the same regardless of which insurer you use. Prices vary among companies, however, so make sure to get quotes from a number of insurers.

Also, don't forget that your right to join a Medigap plan only lasts for six months after enrolling in Part B. After this six-month window, you can (and likely will) be denied Medigap coverage, or you will be charged a higher premium. In some situations (for example, if you move, or if your state grants extra protections) you may be guaranteed the right to sign up for Medigap beyond that six-month window. If not, you can be denied a plan.

How Medigap Plans Are Priced

Insurers that offer Medigap plans have three options when it comes to pricing plans:

• **Issue-Age Rating** Plans priced by issue age set their premiums based on how old you are when you first sign up. Your premium will not rise as you age (with small exceptions, such as accounting for inflation).

• **Community Rating** These plans charge the same amount to everyone enrolled in them, regardless of age. The premiums for these plans also won't rise over time.

• **Attained-Age Rating** Plans priced by attained age will go up each year on your birthday. Premiums may start out quite low, but they can end up becoming more expensive than other plans as you age.

The way insurers rate their plans can greatly affect what you pay. When you ask insurers for a quote, make sure to find out which rating system they use, so you understand whether your premiums will change over time.

You should also ask insurers if they offer discounts for women, nonsmokers or other groups of people. Many do, and those discounts can save you money.

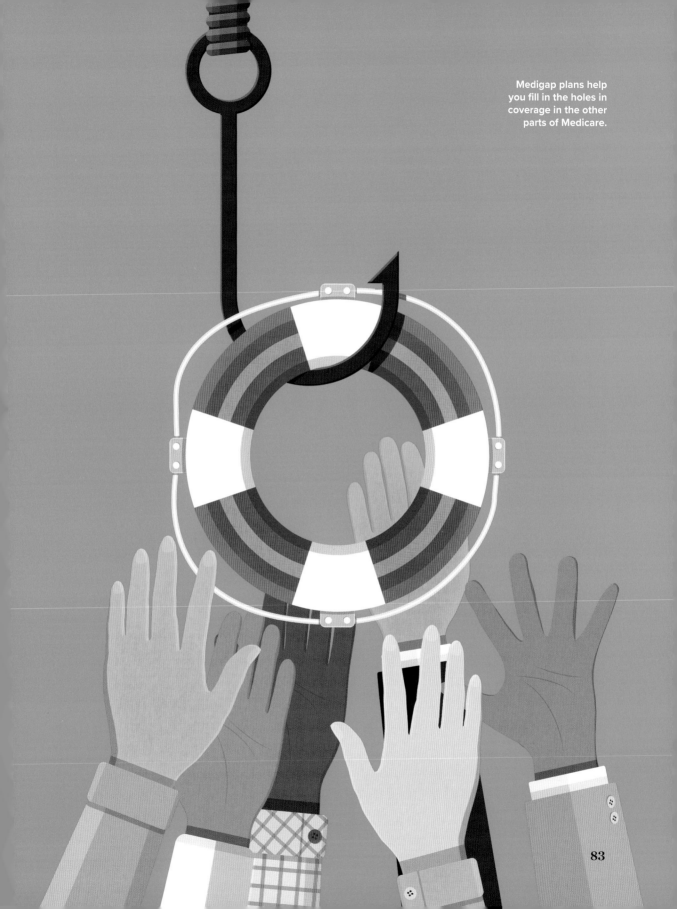

Medigap plans help you fill in the holes in coverage in the other parts of Medicare.

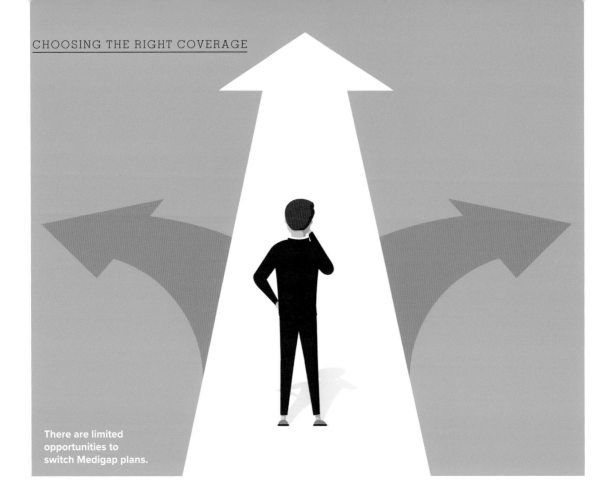

There are limited opportunities to switch Medigap plans.

Which Plan to Choose

Unfortunately, none of us can predict the kind of health care we'll need, or when we'll need it. Ideally, Medicare helps ensure that as you age your costs will never be more than you can pay. For maximum peace of mind (and long-term savings), experts recommend that you spring for the most comprehensive Medigap coverage you can afford. You'll have fewer out-of-pocket costs down the line, and if you ever want to switch between plans, it will be easier to do.

Planning to enroll? Be sure to review your 2020 Medigap options closely. As of Jan. 1, 2020, Medigap plans sold to new Medicare enrollees aren't allowed to cover the Part B deductible. As a result of this, Plans C and F are no longer available as of the beginning of the year. If you were eligible for Medicare before Jan. 1, 2020, but hadn't enrolled, however, you may still be able to buy one of these plans.

Switching Medigap Plans

Generally, it's against the rules to switch Medigap plans each year. However there are some exceptions, and some states do offer protections for those who want to switch. If you're unhappy in Medigap, you can take advantage of the next open enrollment period and switch to a Medicare Advantage plan. When you do so, your first year on Medicare Advantage is considered a trial period—which is particularly useful if you're unsure about how well your plan is working for you. It means if you don't like it, you can switch back to your Medigap policy on the same terms with no penalty. However, this exception only applies the first time you try Medicare Advantage, so you can only take advantage of the opportunity once. ■

GETTING HELP Choosing the right plan can feel overwhelming, but you don't have to go it alone

From Original Medicare and prescription drug coverage to Medigap and Advantage plans, it can be difficult to sift through the various Medicare options. The best fit for you depends on several factors, including your individual medical needs, income, and doctor or hospital preferences. Here are some organizations and resources that can help guide you toward the right decision for your particular circumstances.

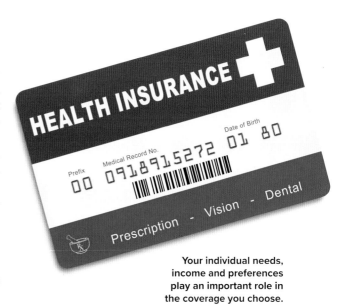

Your individual needs, income and preferences play an important role in the coverage you choose.

Medicare.gov

Medicare.gov offers detailed information about all the parts of Medicare, as well as online tools that can walk you through the questions you should ask when choosing coverage. The tools will help you make the right decision based on cost, the level of coverage you need, and whether you want to keep your current doctors or would be OK with switching. The website can also help explain how Medicare works with other coverage you may have through an employer, a union or the military. If you're curious about Medicare Advantage plans, also known as Medi-

care Part C, you can search for and view details of the plans on this site.

State Health Insurance Programs

If you prefer in-person assistance, check out the State Health Insurance Program (SHIP). SHIP provides free, personalized health insurance counseling to Medicare-eligible individuals, their families and caregivers. The program is staffed by highly trained volunteers who can guide you through the process of choosing and paying for your Medicare coverage and answer your questions. A SHIP counselor can help you apply for a Medicare Savings Program, review health and prescription drug plans and explain how Medicare works with supplemental policies, retiree coverage, Medicaid and other insurers.

SHIP counselors are volunteers—they don't get any payments from insurance companies or doctors' offices. Their main concern is your best interest, so you don't have to worry that the advice they give you isn't objective. To connect with a local SHIP counselor, visit shiptacenter.org or give the SHIP locator a call at 877-839-2675.

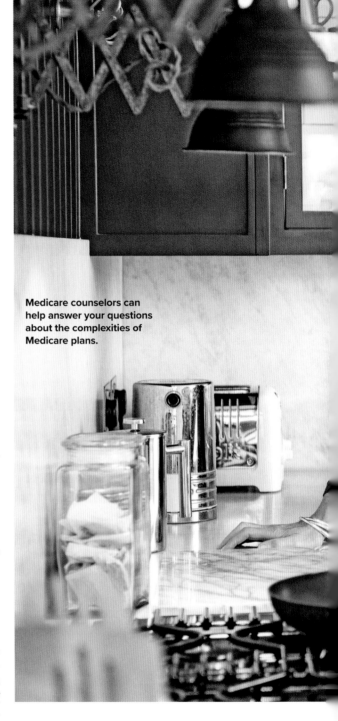

Medicare counselors can help answer your questions about the complexities of Medicare plans.

The Medicare Rights Center

The Medicare Rights Center is a national non-profit consumer rights organization that can also help you and your family navigate the complexities of Medicare. The organization offers many resources and programs, including a national helpline where volunteers and staff provide direct assistance in understanding Medicare benefits and finding the right coverage. You can call the Medicare Rights Helpline at 800-333-4114. At medicarerights.org, you can also sign up for free email newsletters and alerts that will keep you up to date on the latest Medicare news.

Using all the Medicare resources available to you can help you find plans that match your needs and get answers to your important questions.

Additional Options

You can also go to an insurance agent or broker for help choosing a Medicare plan. Agents and brokers offer a wealth of information and experience—they must be licensed in the state where they work and complete annual training sessions to expand their knowledge of Medicare.

When you are working with an agent or a broker to find a plan, it's important to remember that they are compensated for enrolling consumers in certain policies. In other words, they may

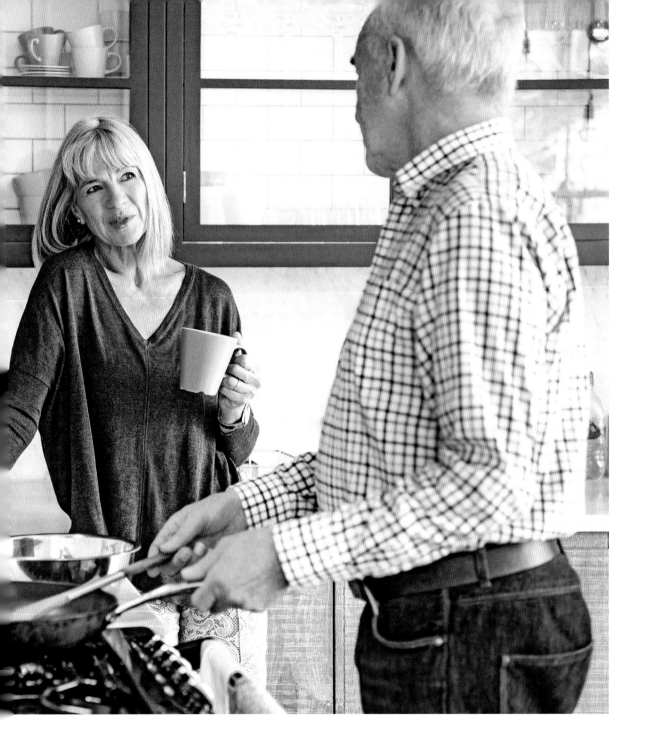

have a conflict of interest in what they are rec-ommending—so you'll want to find someone you trust who can be objective and keep your best interests in mind. You can find more de-tailed information about agent and broker com-pensation for any plan that you may be interest-ed in at the Centers for Medicare & Medicaid website, cms.gov. ∎

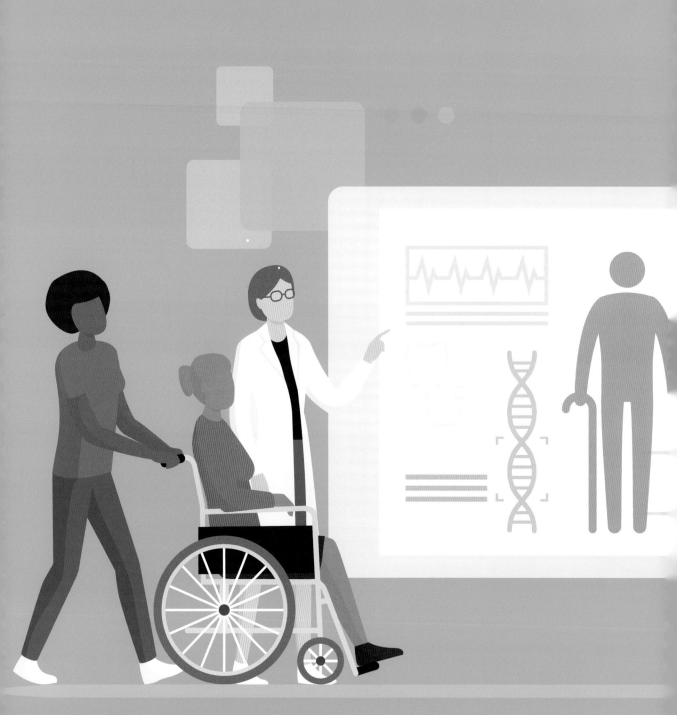

Using Your Plan

Getting the most out of Medicare

GETTING STARTED WITH MEDICARE You've got a plan that works for you. Now what?

You may think choosing your plan is the end of your Medicare-related paperwork, but there are still a few more steps you'll need to take before you can start receiving benefits.

Understanding Your Medicare Cards

Once you enroll in any type of Medicare plan, the government sends you a Medicare card. It's red, white and blue and specifies if you're enrolled in Part A, Part B or both. You'll receive this card no matter which type of coverage you choose: Original Medicare or Medicare Advantage (MA). However, if you've enrolled in any kind of private insurance plan, such as Medicare Advantage, Medigap or Part D, you'll receive an additional card from that plan's company.

If you're on Original Medicare, you'll show your Medicare card when paying for care (as well as your Medigap card, if you have one). If you enrolled in Part D,

The government's mymedicare.gov site makes keeping track of your health care records convenient, but only if you sign up for an account.

the company that issues your Part D coverage will send you yet another card, which you'll need to show when you go to the pharmacy.

If you have Medicare Advantage, you'll show your MA plan's card for any care or when filling your prescriptions, if your plan includes drug coverage. Keep your government-issued Medicare card handy as well, in case a provider asks to see it.

Online First Steps

• **Authorization Forms** You are the only person who can legally get your personal health information from Medicare. If you want someone else, like a family member, to be able to speak to Medicare on your behalf, you need to fill out an authorization form, available on the government's Medicare website (medicare.gov).

• **Sign Up Online** The government provides 24-hour access to your claims, eligibility information, deductible status and lots of other helpful information online through mymedicare.gov. The service makes keeping track of your health care records super convenient—but only if you take the time to sign up for an account.

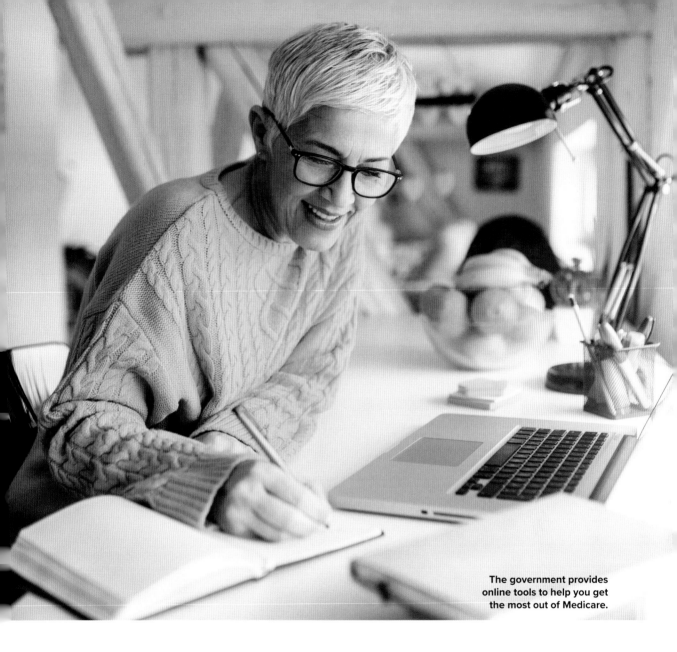

The government provides online tools to help you get the most out of Medicare.

• **Understand What's Covered** The government's website also provides thorough lists and explanations of what Medicare covers and what it doesn't. The tool can also help you anticipate the cost of services you may need in the future.

Wellness Visits

During your first 12 months on Medicare, you definitely should take advantage of the initial "Welcome to Medicare" preventive doctor's office visit. This consultation is free, and your Part B deductible doesn't apply. It's essentially a checkup during which the doctor will perform some basic examinations to get a picture of your overall health. You're also entitled to an annual wellness visit, during which your doctor can recommend specific steps you can take to stay healthy, as well as any health issues you should keep an eye on. ∎

FINANCIAL ASSISTANCE AND OTHER HELP
How to access aid when your premiums and other costs are too high

Medicare is supposed to keep health care affordable for seniors. But if you're on a fixed income, monthly premiums can be a burden, especially if you're paying for care that you're not using. Luckily, you've got options if you need help covering your premiums. Most vary by state, so make sure to research the programs available in your area.

Medicare Advantage
You'll always pay a premium for Part B, but some MA plans don't charge additional premiums on top of that. Since many MA plans also cover prescription drugs, vision, hearing and dental care, a zero-premium MA plan may be your best option for keeping your monthly payments low, depending on your income. Just keep in mind that these premium-free plans may have high deductibles.

Medicaid
More than one in five Medicare beneficiaries is also on Medicaid. Medicaid is the government program that provides health insurance to low-income people. Each state sets its own Medicaid guidelines, so you'll need to check with your local social services office to determine if you're eligible. Those eligible for both Medicare and Medicaid are known as "dual eligible." When you enroll in both Medicare and Medicaid, Medicare is your primary insurer, meaning that it pays its share first. Medicaid then pays for additional costs (such as your coinsurance and deductible). It's also worth noting that Medicaid also covers certain services Medicare does not, such as personal care and long-term care services.

Medicare Savings Programs
Many dual-eligible patients will be automatically enrolled in a Medicare Savings Program (MSP). There are four types of MSPs. Each has a different income limit for qualification, and different benefits. The income limits apply nationwide—they don't vary by state. The four different types are:

•**Qualified Medicare Beneficiary (QMB, often pronounced "Quimby")** This MSP pays your premiums for Parts A and B. Generally, if you have QMB

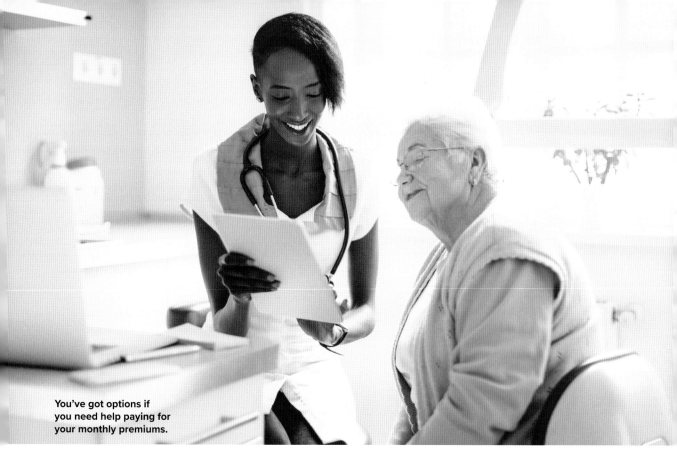

You've got options if you need help paying for your monthly premiums.

you won't be billed for services covered by Medicare as long as your provider participates in the program.

• **Specified Low-Income Medicare Beneficiary (SLMB)** This MSP only pays Part B premiums.

• **Qualifying Individual (QI) Program** This MSP also pays only for your Part B premium. It has a higher income and resource limit than the SLMB, so it's a little easier to qualify for.

• **Qualified Disabled and Working Individuals (QDWI)** This MSP pays the Part A premium for disabled individuals who are returning to work and are no longer entitled to premium-free Part A.

MSPs have other benefits in addition to covering a premium. Enrollment in an MSP qualifies you for full Extra Help, which supplements your Part D drug coverage. And an MSP will cover any penalties you owe for delaying enrollment in Part B.

Extra Help

Extra Help is a program administered by the Social Security Administration (not Medicare) that is designed to provide assistance to people with limited income and resources in helping to pay for their prescriptions. You can apply for Extra Help even if you don't already have drug coverage. If you're approved, you'll need to enroll in a Part D plan, and your Extra Help benefits will be applied to that plan. Extra Help has five different levels, which offer varying amounts of assistance based upon your income level and assets. If you qualify for full Extra Help (level one of the four available), you will have zero out-of-pocket expenses for your medications. With partial Extra Help, you will still have some out-of-pocket costs, but they will be much lower than they would be otherwise. Another benefit: No matter what level of Extra Help you qualify for, you won't have to worry about falling into the donut hole. ∎

USING YOUR HSA Maximize your health care savings to pay your medical expenses

Getting Medicare coverage doesn't mean saying goodbye to all health care costs. The money that's been piling up in your health savings account (HSA) can go a long way toward paying for health services Medicare doesn't cover, as well as copayments, coinsurance and deductibles. You can even use funds from your HSA to pay premiums for Part A, Part B, Part D and Medicare Advantage plans. The only premiums you can't pay tax-free are Medigap premiums.

How HSAs Work

HSAs are specialized savings accounts designed to offer a tax-free way to cover out-of-pocket medical expenses. As with a 401(k) or traditional IRA, contributions are made pre-tax (or are tax deductible if made outside of payroll deductions), then grow tax-free.

But unlike those other plans, with an HSA you can always make tax-free withdrawals to pay for qualified medical expenses such as doctor's office visit copays, prescription drugs and dental visits—even eyeglasses and medical travel. In fact, your HSA account typically comes with a debit card you can use to pay those bills.

You can use HSA funds to pay for current medical costs—which are effectively discounted, since every dollar spent hasn't been reduced by taxes. If you accumulate those savings over the years in a diverse portfolio, you'll have a great way to offset some of your medical expenses in retirement.

No More HSA Contributions

To be eligible to contribute to an HSA, you have to have a high-deductible insurance plan. These plans carry much higher out-of-pocket costs than most other plans—often more than the annual HSA contribution limit. On the other hand, they typically have smaller monthly premiums.

Medicare does not count as a high-deductible insurance plan. That means you won't be able to make any more contributions to your HSA once you're covered by Medicare. Keep this fact in mind as you approach your retirement age—it may make

It may make sense to max out your contributions to your HSA while you're still working to ensure you add as much as possible while you can.

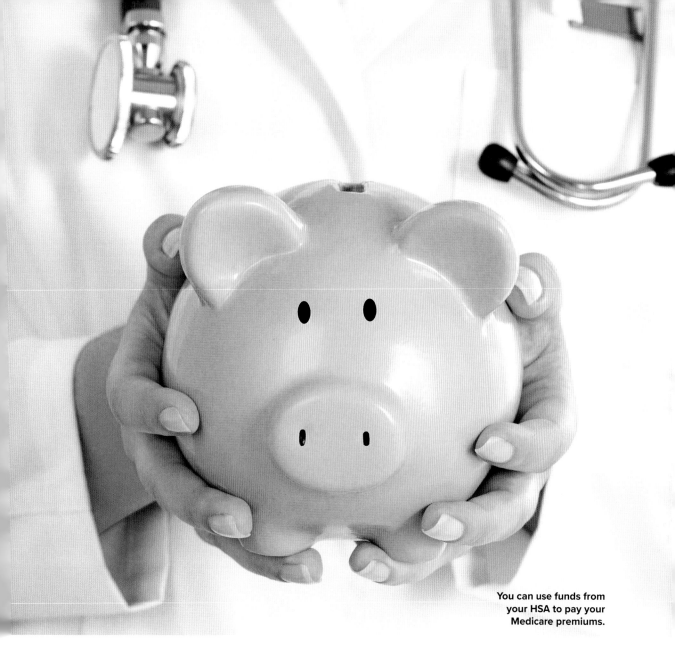

You can use funds from your HSA to pay your Medicare premiums.

sense to max out your contributions while you are still working to make sure you add as much money as possible to your account while you still can.

What Happens If You've Saved More Than You Can Spend?

Once you turn 65, you can withdraw your HSA savings for any reason without any penalties whatsoever—you will just end up having to pay taxes on withdrawals that don't pay for health care–related expenses, though withdrawals for health expenses continue to be tax free.

If you wind up with more in your HSA than you can spend on health care–related expenses, you can simply make withdrawals and pay the related taxes. You can even assign the account to a beneficiary and pass it along as an inheritance. ■

MAKING THE MOST OF YOUR MEDICARE BENEFITS Stay well-informed and get the care you deserve

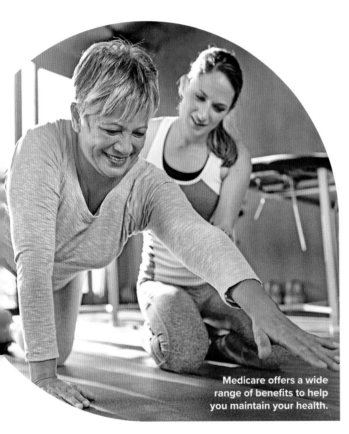

Medicare offers a wide range of benefits to help you maintain your health.

Once you're enrolled in Medicare, you will become entitled to a range of benefits beyond what you'll get at the doctor's office. Knowing what's involved and how to the most of them will help you stay healthy and keep your benefits working for you.

Know Your Benefits

All Medicare plans entitle you to a free annual wellness visit, which can help nip potential health issues in the bud. If you're on a Part C plan, you may also have access to additional benefits that Original Medicare doesn't cover, such as vision, hearing and dental care. Some plans even cover the cost of gym memberships, fitness classes and online brain games to keep your mind healthy.

Exercise Your Right to Appeal

Your doctor assured you that your latest appointments would be covered. So why is Medicare denying your claim? It could be a clerical error, or it could be based on a belief that your care wasn't

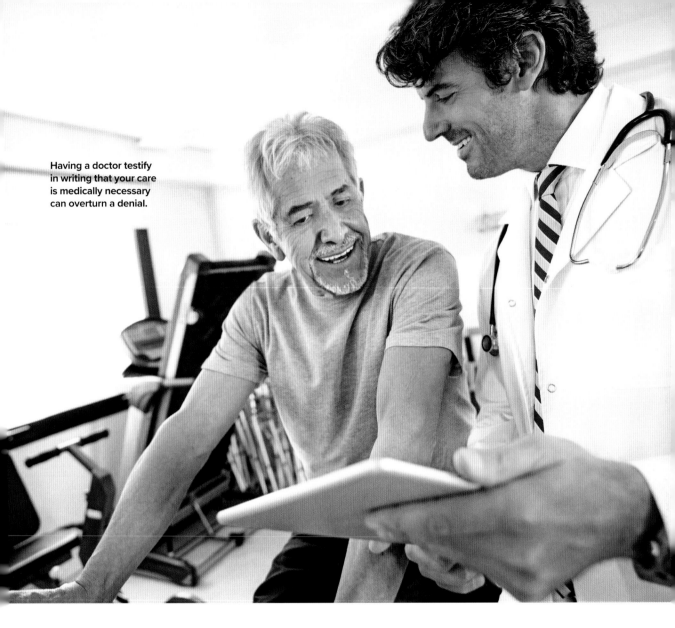

Having a doctor testify in writing that your care is medically necessary can overturn a denial.

medically necessary. Regardless of the reason, don't take an initial "no" for an answer when it comes to getting your care covered. In many cases, having your doctor testify (in writing) that a service or specific prescription was medically necessary is enough to overturn a denial.

Get Professional Help

If you need help submitting an appeal, contact your state's State Health Insurance Assistance Program (SHIP). Every state has one. These programs provide free counseling about all things Medicare, from understanding eligibility to switching plans. And they can help you fight a denial. SHIPs can also help keep your support network well-informed by educating family members and caregivers about Medicare. SHIP counseling is an important resource. It's not paid for by an insurance company or health care provider; it's unbiased counseling with your best interests in mind. ∎

USING YOUR PART D COVERAGE What to know before you walk into the pharmacy

Getting your prescriptions filled should be hassle-free. But that's not always the case. Things will go more smoothly if you make sure to bring the right documents with you and call your health care provider for backup when necessary. The following tips can help:

Using Part D for the First Time

• Know When Your Coverage Begins Generally, your Part D coverage goes into effect on the first day of the month after you enrolled in your plan. If you enrolled or switched plans during open enrollment (Oct. 15 to Dec. 7), your coverage will begin Jan. 1. Either way, you will receive your Part D card in the mail before your coverage goes into effect, but you will not be able to use it until your coverage actually starts.

> ⬇
> Many Part D plans offer convenient mail-order prescription services, some of which offer extras like discounts on drugs and free shipping.

• Know Which Pharmacies Are Covered Before you have your doctor call in a prescrip-tion, make sure that your pharmacy is in your plan's network.

• Have Your Documents Ready
When you show up to the pharmacy, you'll need a few pieces of documentation: your official Medicare card (the one sent to you by the government), as well as a government-issued photo ID and your card for your Part D plan. If you have Medicaid or Extra Help, you will also need to bring proof of coverage in those programs in order to receive their benefits.

Different Ways to Get Your Drugs
Trekking to your local pharmacy may not be the most convenient way to get your medications. Many Part D plans have mail-order services for prescriptions. Some even offer a discount on mail-order drugs, and all should include free shipping. While mail-order prescriptions can be extremely convenient if you live in a rural area or have difficulty leaving the house, there are a few things to keep in mind:

• Generally, you can only order a 90-day (three-month) supply of medication at one time—so this

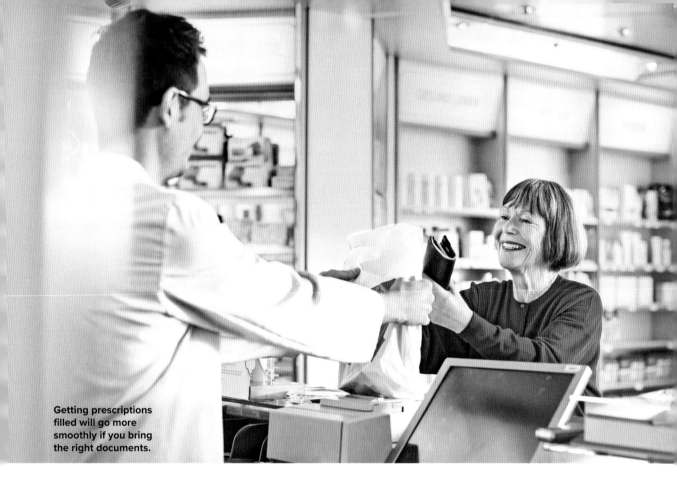

Getting prescriptions filled will go more smoothly if you bring the right documents.

option usually works best for medications you take on a regular basis.

• Buying three months' worth of medication at a time means you'll spend more at once than you would if you were purchasing it month by month. As a result, you may end up in the donut hole slightly faster than you would if you paid for your medications one month at a time.

• You'll need to request refills over the phone or online—they won't be automatically mailed to you. Since delivery can take seven to 10 days, waiting until the last minute could leave you stuck without the medications you need for a week or more.

If mail-order meds aren't for you, you can still use your local in-network pharmacy. However, for medications that require special care, such

as some cancer medications, you'll need to go to a specialty pharmacy preferred by your plan. If there isn't a preferred specialty pharmacy in your area, call your plan to arrange an exception so that you can visit a local pharmacy even if it's normally out of network.

Long-term care facilities—for example, nursing homes—generally have in-house pharmacies that dispense meds in individual doses. If you move into a facility and its pharmacy isn't in your plan's network, call your plan ASAP. When you first enter a nursing home, your plan is required to cover any drugs you're already on for at least 90 days. You're also entitled to switch Part D plans immediately upon entering a nursing home, with no need to wait for open enrollment—so if your plan won't work with your facility's pharmacy in the long run, you can switch to one that will.

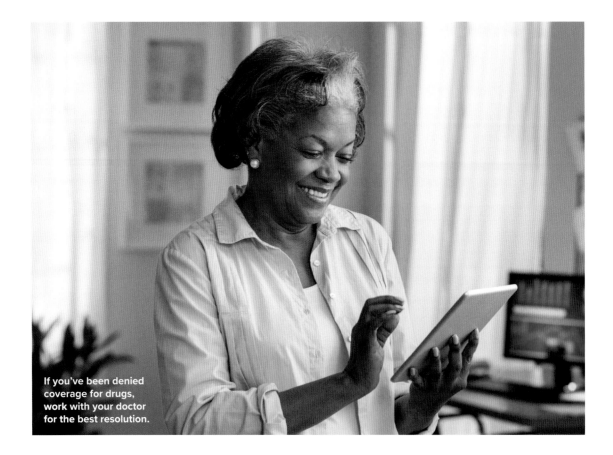

If you've been denied coverage for drugs, work with your doctor for the best resolution.

When Your Plan Won't Pay

Picture this: You show up at the pharmacy to pick up your drugs, but the pharmacist tells you they're not covered by your plan. What happened? Part D plans have the right to restrict coverage for drugs in their formularies if they believe the drug could pose a safety risk (think opioids), if your doctor has prescribed a higher dosage than is typical or if the plan covers a comparable (but less-expensive) drug that you haven't tried.

Finding out that your meds aren't covered is frustrating—and it can potentially pose a serious health risk. If you find yourself in this situation, you need to request an exception.

Requesting an exception is technically known as requesting a coverage determination. In practi-

cal terms, it means filling out the necessary form on Medicare's website declaring which medication you need and why it is medically necessary. You'll have a much better chance of getting an exception if your doctor or someone from their office submits the form on your behalf.

Your plan will have 72 hours to respond to your request after you submit it. If waiting that long is potentially life-threatening, your doctor can demand an expedited exception, which gives your plan only 24 hours to respond. If your exception is denied, you have the right to appeal that decision—known as asking for reconsideration. If this effort fails, there are even higher levels of appeal you can turn to—all the way up to the Federal District Court—but in many cases it won't come to that. ∎

COMMON MEDICARE MISHAPS Avoid mistakes to get the most out of your coverage

Medicare's maze of rules and regulations can make it easy to miss the fine print; this can result in costly mistakes. Avoiding the following common errors will help ensure you have access to the coverage you're entitled to.

Assuming You're Automatically Signed Up When You Turn 65

Although you become eligible for Medicare when you turn 65, only people receiving Social Security or railroad retirement benefits when they turn 65 are automatically enrolled in Medicare Parts A and B. If you aren't in that group, you'll need to actively enroll in Medicare during your initial enrollment period. You can do so by visiting a local Social Security office, calling Social Security at 800-772-1213, or going online at ssa.gov.

If you don't sign up when you first become eligible, you'll end up paying penalties when you try to sign up later. If you're still working and have an employer or union group health insurance plan, you can delay signing up for Part B without penalty as long as you eventually sign up within eight months after you leave your job. If you wait too long to sign up for Part B, you might be stuck waiting for the next enrollment period (January through March every year).

Not Taking Advantage of Open Enrollment

Whether you initially enroll in Original Medicare or an Advantage plan, you aren't stuck with that plan forever. You can choose a new plan during the annual Medicare open enrollment period from Oct. 15 through Dec. 7. Plans can change over the years, and you may wind up missing out on cheaper alternatives if you don't shop around.

The open enrollment period is also a good time to reassess your Part D prescription drug coverage. It's not uncommon for these plans to change from year to year, so it's important to re-evaluate and make sure your plan still meets your needs.

You can view, research and compare Advantage and Part D plans using the Medicare Plan Finder tool on medicare.gov/find-a-plan.

101

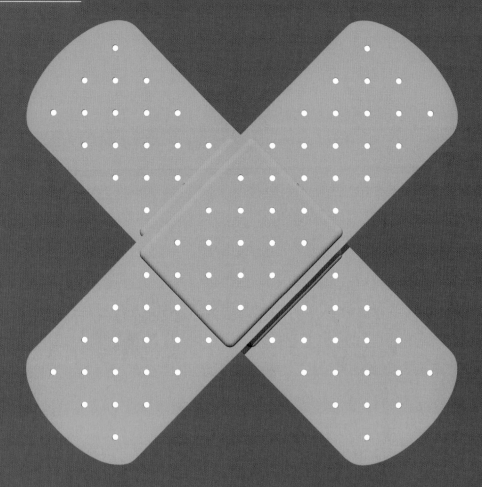

When choosing a plan, consider what coverage you may need down the road.

Failing to Plan for the Future

No one has a crystal ball, but when choosing a Medicare plan it's important to consider what coverage you may eventually need in addition to addressing any health conditions you currently have. This is especially true when choosing a Medicare supplement or Medigap policy.

You might not think about Medigap plans until you are facing large out-of-pocket costs or need additional coverage not included in Original Medicare. But if you wait too long, insurers can reject you or charge you more based on your medical history.

If you think you may eventually need services Original Medicare doesn't cover (like hearing aids, dental care or vision care), you may want to shop around for a Medicare Advantage plan that covers those extra services. ∎

MEDICARE FRAUD
What it looks like and how to avoid it

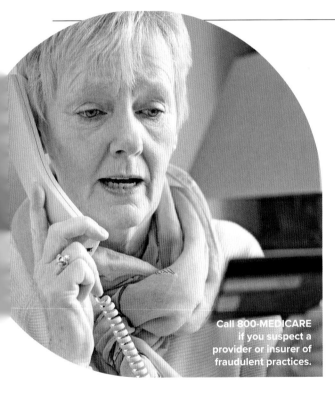

Call 800-MEDICARE if you suspect a provider or insurer of fraudulent practices.

cost the system more than $52 billion in 2017. The government combats fraudulent practices through a network of regional strike forces, but believe it or not, you can also play a part in the fight against fraud.

Fraudulent Billing Practices

One of the most common forms of Medicare fraud involves health care providers who bill for unnecessary services—or even procedures they don't actually perform. Look carefully at the items on your Medicare Summary Notice—if there are services and charges that don't look familiar, your provider may be committing fraud.

The complexity of Medicare—the overwhelming amount of paperwork, obscure jargon, acronyms and government rules and regulations—makes it ripe for fraud and abuse. This is a big problem: the Government Accountability Office estimates that Medicare fraud

Sometimes, unscrupulous providers steal personal Medicare information and use it to get paid for services they never delivered. Take extra care to keep your personal and Medicare registration information secure. Think of your Medicare card like a credit card and only share it when absolutely necessary. Generally speak-

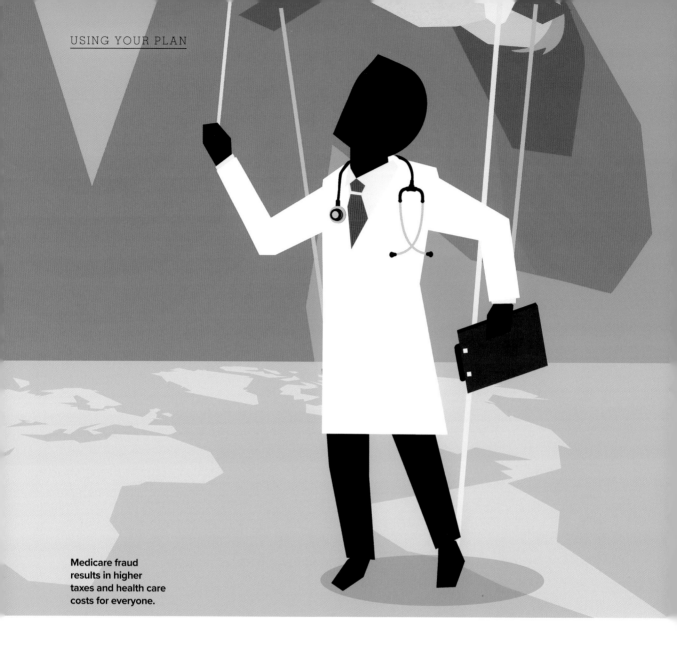

Medicare fraud results in higher taxes and health care costs for everyone.

ing, no one (other than your providers' office staffs) needs to see it.

Fraudulent Sales Practices

Another common form of Medicare fraud involves insurance agents selling plans under false pretenses. For example, an agent may tell you a certain Medicare Advantage plan provides services it does not, or they may falsely claim that regulations prevent you from choosing a competitor's plan. Check with the insurance company offering the plan to confirm any dubious claims.

Dealing With Medicare Fraud

Here's how you can help: If you suspect a provider or insurer of fraud, hold onto any documentation that you have and call the Department of Health and Human Services at 800-MEDICARE or the department's Inspector General at 800-HHS-TIPS. ∎

MEDICARE RESOURCES
Learn where you can get help, find in-person assistance and gather more information

Navigating the complex world of Medicare can be confusing for many of us. Luckily, there are a variety of resources available that can provide helpful information on a host of topics, including how to choose the best options for your needs.

General Information
Online resources—like the Centers for Medicare & Medicaid Services (CMS) website, cms.gov, and the Medicare website, medicare.gov—are good places to start for in-depth information on the various components of Medicare and how they work together. These websites offer consumer guides on just about any Medicare topic.

CMS publishes "Medicare & You," a handbook with comprehensive information about plan details and answers to common questions.

The AARP offers several online resources, including a consumer guide to Part D coverage and an archive of common Medicare questions asked by AARP members. Go to AARP's Medicare Resource Center at aarp.org/health.

CMS also publishes "Medicare & You," a handbook that contains comprehensive information on Medicare, from eligibility requirements and enrollment periods to frequently asked questions. The agency updates the handbook annually and mails a copy to each Medicare recipient in the fall. You can also download an electronic copy at mymedicare.gov.

Patricia Barry's book *Medicare for Dummies* is another useful resource. She spells out in clear, step-by-step instructions how and when to enroll, how to find the right plan for you, ways to avoid costly mistakes and tips for reducing your out-of-pocket expenses.

Claims and Appeals
For detailed information on your rights and protections as a Medicare beneficiary, visit medicare.gov/claims-appeals. This section of Medicare's website also provides helpful information on

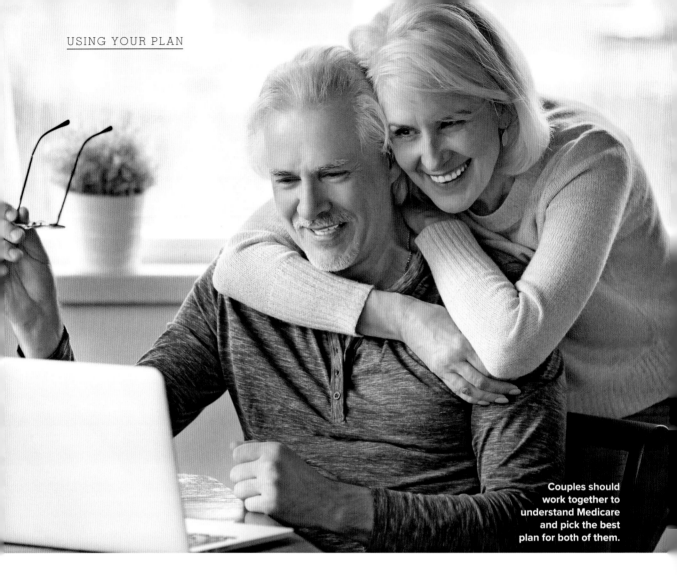

Couples should work together to understand Medicare and pick the best plan for both of them.

how to appeal coverage or payment decisions made by Medicare, how to file a claim for Medicare bills when your provider can't or won't, and how to track the status of your claims.

Details About Plan Options

You can find a list of available health and drug plans in the "Medicare & You" handbook. If you want to dig deeper into the details, visit Medicare's plan finder tool at medicare.gov/find-a-plan. You can use this tool to:

- View a list of covered prescription drugs for each plan
- Find doctors
- View a side-by-side comparison of costs for different plans
- Compare hospitals and pharmacies

Talk to a Real Person

Online resources and books can be useful tools for gathering information, but when it comes to asking questions about your specific circumstances, nothing beats talking to a real person. The organization or agency best suited to assist you depends on what kind of question you have.

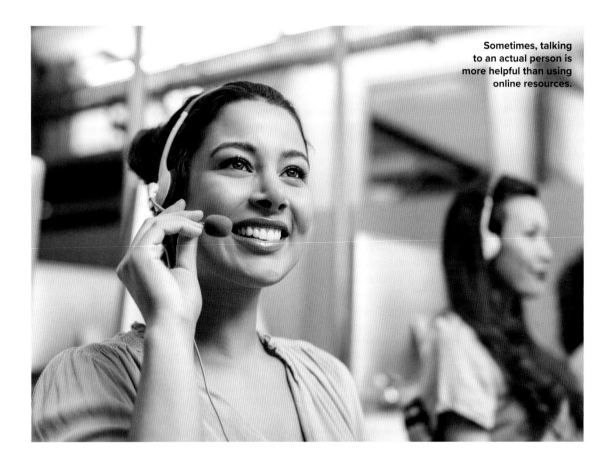

Sometimes, talking to an actual person is more helpful than using online resources.

Contact the Social Security Administration at 800-772-1213 for questions about:

• Medicare eligibility
• Enrolling in Part A or B
• Obtaining a replacement Medicare card

Contact the CMS at 800-663-4227 for questions about:

• Medicare benefits and coverage
• Choosing a Part D drug plan or a Medicare Advantage health plan
• Filing an appeal
• Medicare Savings Programs
• Finding a provider that accepts Medicare patients in your area

When you call CMS, be sure to have your Medicare card available for reference and be prepared to give them your Medicare number.

If you have specific questions about your plan or policy, check your card or plan materials for the right number to call for assistance.

Contact Your State Health Insurance Assistance Program (SHIP)

Your state's SHIP can also help guide you through the Medicare system. SHIPs provide local, personalized counseling and assistance on an array of Medicare topics, including your benefits and coverage, filing appeals and understanding how to use your Medicare plan. Visit shiptacenter.org for the contact information of your local SHIP. ∎

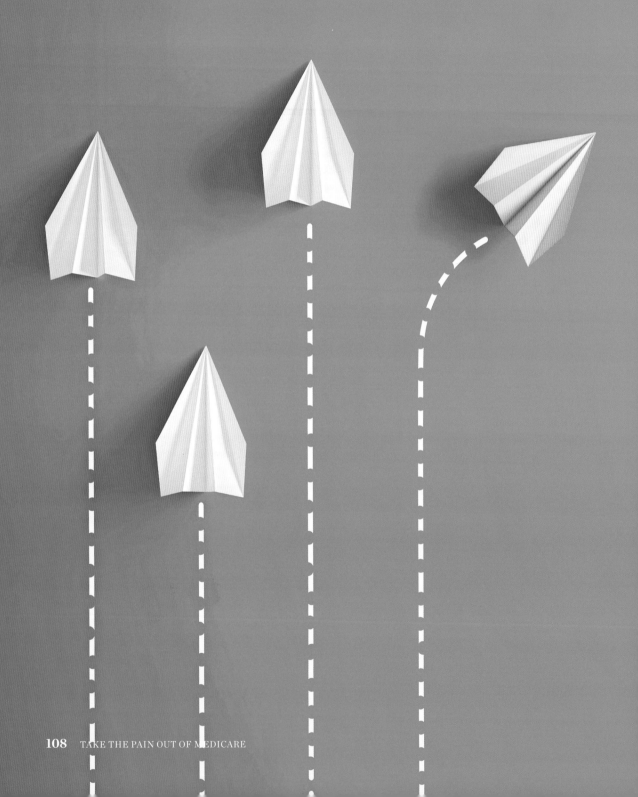

Changing Your Coverage

When your health care needs shift,
it may be time to look for a different plan

HOW TO SWITCH MEDICARE PLANS
Understanding open enrollment, disenrollment and special enrollment periods

No matter how carefully you weigh your options before signing up for Medicare, you still may end up having to change plans at some point. Your health care needs could shift, you could move to a new state, or your income could change dramatically, leaving you with few good options aside from switching plans. Also, your plan itself can change in ways that make it less suitable for you. Medicare has strict rules for when and how you can change plans, so the keys to a successful initial enrollment still apply when you're changing plans: Know your deadlines—and mark your calendar.

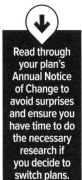

Read through your plan's Annual Notice of Change to avoid surprises and ensure you have time to do the necessary research if you decide to switch plans.

You Love Your Coverage, So Why Change?

If you're happy with your coverage, you don't have to do anything during the government's annual open enrollment period. Your plan generally will renew for the next year (assuming it's not going bankrupt, which does happen occasionally). However, it's very important that you read your plan's Annual Notice of Change (ANOC), which your plan must make sure you receive by Sept. 30. This letter details all of the changes to your plan for the following year. If you haven't received it by the first week of October, contact your plan immediately and ask them to send you a copy.

Most plans make changes every year. And while it may seem tedious to read through them all, doing so can save you a lot of money and frustration. If you don't read your ANOC, you might show up at the pharmacy expecting your usual $10 copay only to find that it's gone up to $85. Read your ANOC to avoid surprises and decide whether the changes make switching plans a good idea.

Open Enrollment: Changing Plans

If you want to alter your Medicare coverage in some way, chances are you will need to do so during open enrollment, which takes place each year from Oct. 15 to Dec. 7. During open enrollment you can:

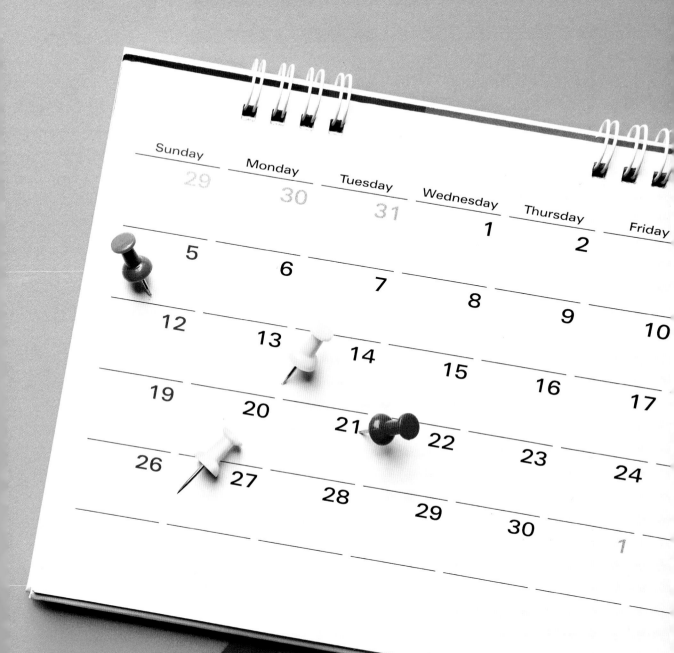

Sunday	Monday	Tuesday	Wednesday	Thursday	Friday
29	30	31	1	2	
5	6	7	8	9	10
12	13	14	15	16	17
19	20	21	22	23	24
26	27	28	29	30	1

You can change plans during open enrollment, which runs Oct. 15 through Dec. 7 yearly.

- Switch from Original Medicare to Medicare Advantage
- Switch between Medicare Advantage plans
- Switch Part D plans
- Sign up for Part D for the first time
- Switch from Medicare Advantage to Original Medicare

When you switch plans during the open enrollment period, your current coverage will remain in place until Jan. 1, after which your new coverage will begin.

Disenrollment

If you're enrolled in a Medicare Advantage plan but want to switch to Original Medicare, you can do so during open enrollment. But you can also take advantage of the separate Medicare Advantage disenrollment period (MADP), which lasts from Jan. 1 to Feb. 14 each year. Your new coverage will begin either Feb. 1 or March 1, depending on when you disenroll.

To start the disenrollment process, call either your MA plan or Medicare directly and request to disenroll. If (and only if) the Medicare Advantage plan you're leaving included Part D coverage, you may use this period to sign up for a Part D plan as well. Since you're switching to Original Medicare, you can also use this period to sign up for a Medigap policy if you wish to do so. However, because this isn't your initial enrollment period, you may be denied Medigap coverage based on your age or health, or the insurance company may charge you a higher premium.

When you change your coverage during open enrollment, your current coverage remains in place until your new coverage starts on Jan. 1.

Special Enrollment

In certain circumstances, you may qualify for a special enrollment period (SEP), during which you can change your Medicare coverage outside of open enrollment. An SEP is based on your personal circumstances, so you may need to do some research to know if your reason for switching care qualifies. It's a good idea to check with your local State Health Insurance Assistance Program (SHIP) to see if your particular situation gives you the option.

Common situations that qualify for an SEP include:

- **Moving Out of Your Plan's Service Area**
This situation relates to MA and Part D plans, which only cover certain geographical areas.

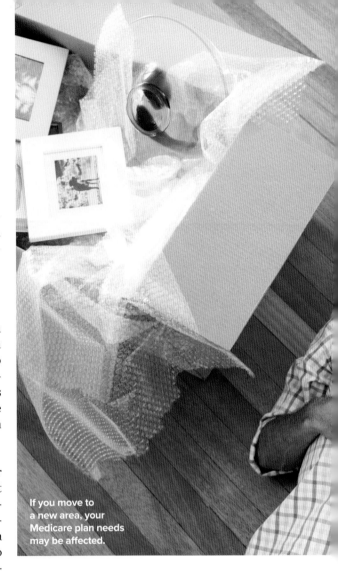

If you move to a new area, your Medicare plan needs may be affected.

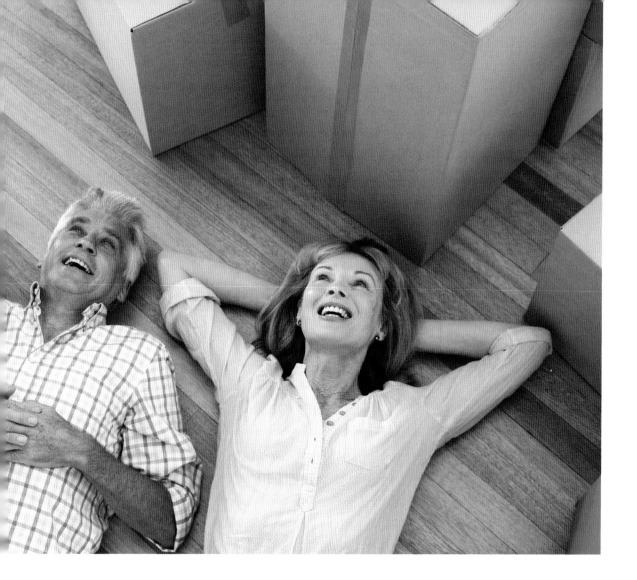

Keep in mind that the criteria for an SEP only apply to permanent moves—not to snowbirding.

• Entering or Leaving a Long-Term Care Facility, Nursing Home or Other Institutional Facility In this situation, the SEP ensures you can find a plan that will work with the facility's pharmacy if your current plan won't provide coverage.

• Contract Violations Committed By Your Plan If your plan doesn't make good on its obligations to you as a beneficiary, you're entitled to an SEP. However, you'll have to contact

Medicare directly to make your case and apply for an SEP.

• Changes to Your Plan That Affect Your Ability to Get Coverage You should receive notice from either Medicare or your insurance company if your plan stops serving your area or stops working with Medicare. If this happens, you're entitled to an SEP so you can find a new plan.

While most SEPs last between two and three months, there's no standard length, and the duration can vary based on a variety of factors. Make sure you know exactly how long yours will last. ■

WHAT TO DO IF A PLAN DROPS YOU
It's unlikely, but you should still be prepared

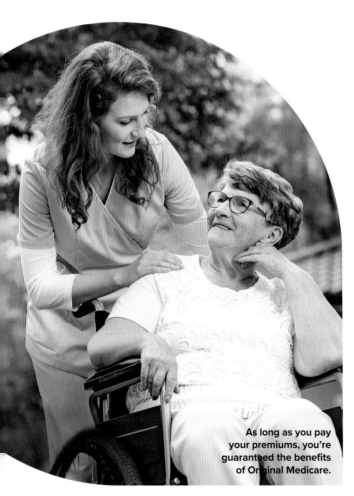

As long as you pay your premiums, you're guaranteed the benefits of Original Medicare.

Medicare guarantees you certain rights. As long as you pay your premiums, you should be guaranteed the right to all of the benefits covered by Original Medicare regardless of your age, your health or where you live. If you abide by Medicare's deadlines (and pay your premiums), you should have access to Part D coverage, Medigap and Medicare Advantage plans as well. However, there are some situations in which you may lose your coverage. Take care to avoid the following:

Failing to Pay Your Premium
Original Medicare is meant to be accessible. Many people are enrolled automatically and have their premiums automatically deducted from their Social Security payments. However, if for any reason you do stop paying your premiums, you will eventually lose your coverage. You'll receive multiple notices that your bill is overdue, and finally (about four months after your initial missed payment) Medicare will be able to drop your coverage.

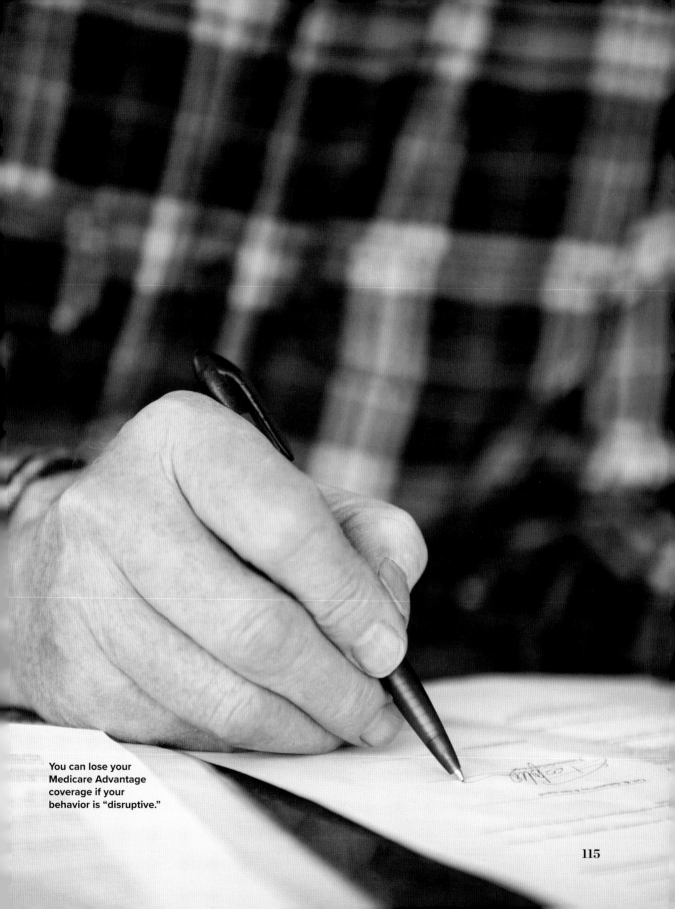

You can lose your
Medicare Advantage
coverage if your
behavior is "disruptive."

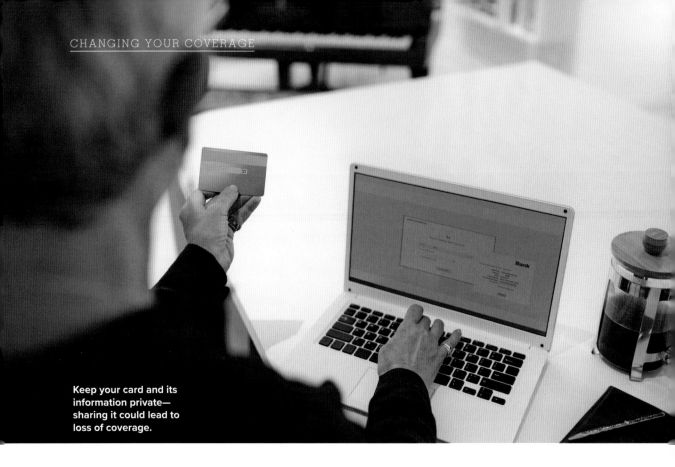

Keep your card and its information private—sharing it could lead to loss of coverage.

When this happens, you also lose eligibility for Part D. You can re-enroll, but you'll need to wait until general enrollment (Jan. 1 to March 31) to sign up—and your coverage won't begin until July. Plus, you'll probably be stuck with higher premiums as a penalty for late enrollment.

Keep in mind that missing any income-related monthly adjustment amounts you owe on Part B or Part D can also lead to loss of coverage.

> To keep your Medicare privileges safe, simply pay your premiums, be honest, ask questions if necessary and don't let others use your card to obtain care.

Committing Medicare Fraud

Medicare fraud can take many forms, including misrepresenting other coverage you have (such as insurance through an employer) or even allowing someone else to use your Medicare card to access care. The simplest ways to avoid losing your coverage: Be honest, ask questions and don't let others use your card to obtain care.

"Disruptive Behavior"

Though Medicare doesn't go into specifics, you can lose your MA coverage if you behave in a way that "substantially impairs" the plan's ability to do its job—namely, providing services to you and/or other beneficiaries. While this possibility may sound scary, MA plans must follow specific steps before they can drop you for this reason. MA plans must also provide reasonable accommodations for beneficiaries with mental illness and developmental disabilities, so this particular clause can't be used to discriminate based on cognitive conditions. If your MA plan does attempt to disenroll you for disruptive behavior, it must also inform you of your right to file a griev-

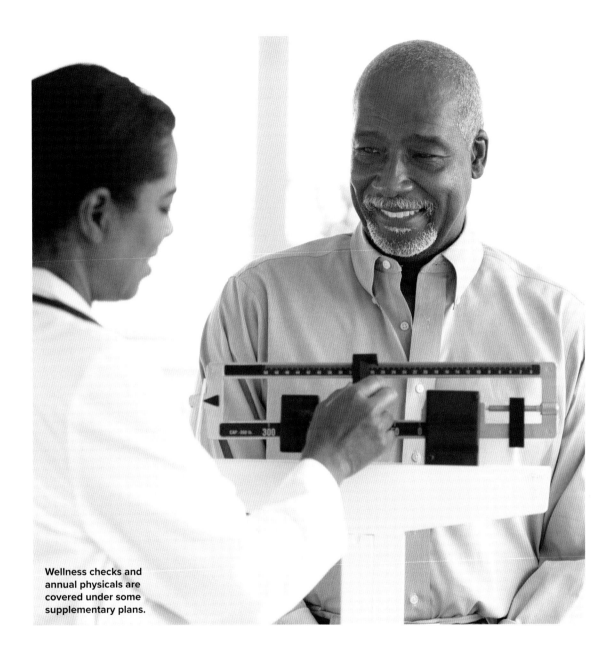

Wellness checks and annual physicals are covered under some supplementary plans.

ance. If your MA plan does ultimately drop you, you'll be put back onto Original Medicare.

What Happens if Your Plan Closes Up Shop
If your insurance company goes bankrupt or decides to stop dealing with Medicare, you'll lose that plan's coverage. However, you'll receive notice from your insurance company or from Medicare beforehand. You'll be entitled to a special enrollment period during which you can select a new plan that will kick in when your old plan ends. Your Medicare Advantage, Part D and Medigap coverage get the same protection. ∎

WHAT TO THINK ABOUT AT RENEWAL TIME
Things to consider when holiday shopping includes searching for new health coverage

Open enrollment happens every year from Oct. 15 to Dec. 7. And while you may be perfectly happy with your Medicare coverage, it's still important to take time to review your benefits and consider whether you want to change plans for the coming year. While you may not like the idea of having to compare plans annually (shouldn't once be enough?), doing so could save you money—and more than a few headaches.

As renewal time draws near, focus on the three C's: coverage, cost and care. That is, make sure your health care needs (including drugs) are covered, at a price you can afford and from providers you trust. Simple, right?

What's Not Changing
Benefits you receive from Original Medicare won't generally change from year to year, because they're determined by the government. Likewise, if you have a Medigap policy, your benefits won't change, either. Medigap plans themselves are also standardized by the government, even though they're provided by private insurers. Your premiums for Original Medicare and Medigap won't go up beyond the rate of inflation unless:

• **Your Income Goes Up** A higher income could affect whether you pay an income-related monthly adjustment amount for Part B.

• **Your Medigap Policy Premium Is Based on Attained-Age** If so, your premium will go up each year on your birthday—but if you did your homework, this increase shouldn't come as a surprise.

Original Medicare and Medigap policies can be used anywhere in the country, so if you move or you're a snowbird, you'll still be covered, no matter where you are. For both Original Medicare and Medigap, there's no need to renew your plan each year—your coverage will continue unchanged as long as you pay your premiums.

What Can Change
Part D plans and Medicare Advantage (MA) plans make changes fairly frequently. Any changes for

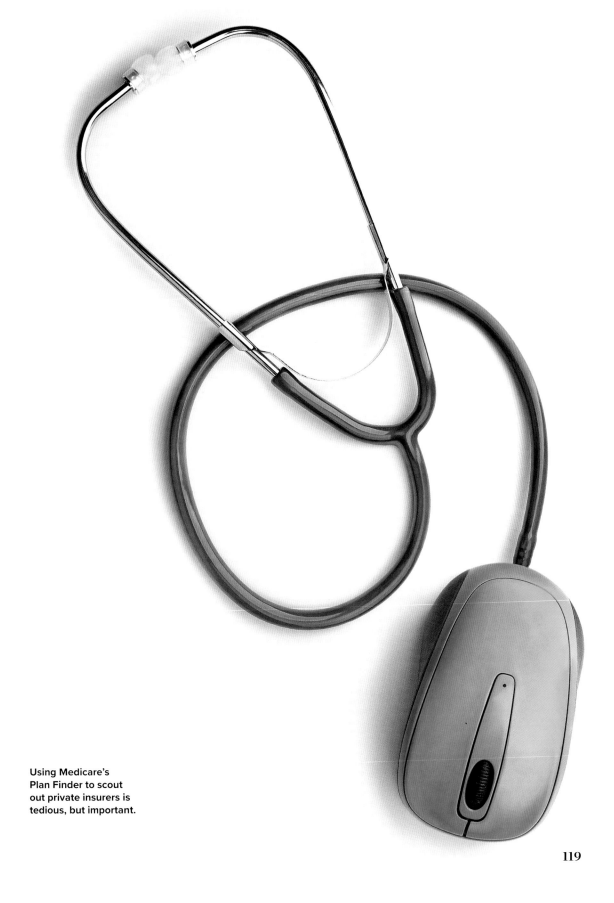

Using Medicare's Plan Finder to scout out private insurers is tedious, but important.

the coming year must be detailed in your plan's Annual Notice of Change (ANOC), which you'll receive by the end of September. If you haven't received it by the beginning of October, call your plan and request one immediately, so you'll have plenty of time to review it.

There may be changes to:

- Your Part D formulary
- Your Part D pharmacy network
- Your MA plan's provider network
- Your MA plan's policies
- Your premiums or deductibles for MA or Part D

Your plan's willingness to grant you an exception for specific drug coverage can also change. Just because your plan made an exception to cover a drug outside of its formulary this year doesn't mean it has to do so next year. Call your plan to ask whether or not you'll need to reapply for the exception. If plan administrators are going to make it difficult to get the drugs you need, you may be better off switching plans while you have the opportunity.

Back to the Plan Finder

Using Medicare's Plan Finder (medicare.gov /find-a-plan)—the online tool provided by the government that helps you find a private insurer—can seem tedious at first. However, you'll likely find that the process gets easier as you get used to it. Even if it doesn't, using it is still worth the time and effort.

Because even if your plan's ANOC doesn't detail any changes that could affect you, other plans may have made changes that could make them a better option. For example, a new insurance company could have entered your area, offering a comparable plan to yours but with a much lower premium or deductible. If you don't bother to check the Plan Finder, you may never hear about new, more attractive options.

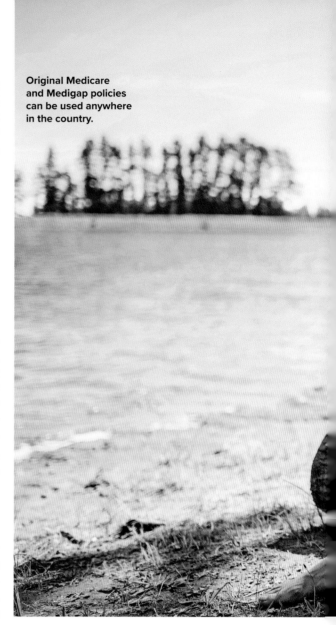

Original Medicare and Medigap policies can be used anywhere in the country.

Switching from Medigap to Medicare Advantage

If until now you've had Original Medicare with a Medigap plan, you may be considering switching to a Medicare Advantage plan for additional benefits, or perhaps to limit your out-of-pocket expenses. However, be careful if you decide to take this step, because once you leave Medigap, you may not be able to get it back. Always check the Plan Finder to avoid unpleasant surprises.

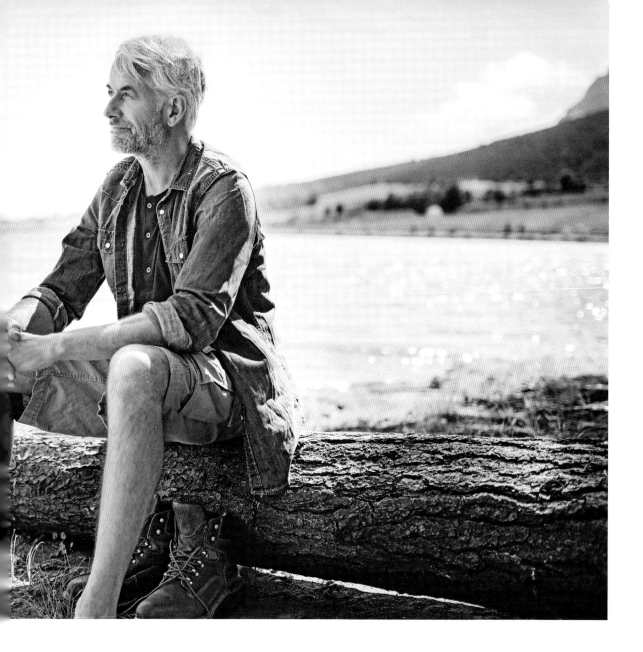

Be aware that if you drop a Medigap policy:

• Your first 12 months in your new MA plan are considered a "trial period." During this trial period, you can still switch back to your original Medigap plan with the same benefits and the same government protections that you had previously.

• This special protection only applies the first time that you switch from Medigap to Medicare Advantage. And it only applies if you already had a Medigap policy. You can't take advantage of this trial period if you're simply going from Original Medicare (with no Medigap) to MA.

• After this 12-month trial period, you no longer have the guaranteed right to a Medigap plan and you may also be denied one in the future. However, you will still be able to switch between Medicare Advantage plans. ■

CHANGING MEDIGAP PLANS It's not always easy, but it's certainly possible

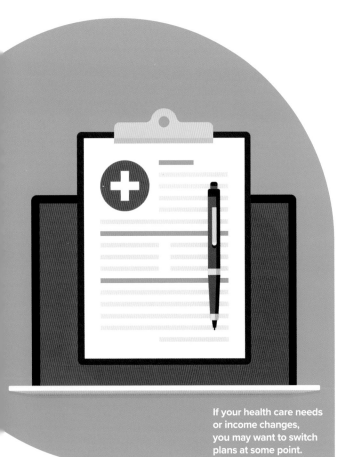

If your health care needs or income changes, you may want to switch plans at some point.

If you enrolled in a Medigap policy during your initial six-month window, your plan is guaranteed renewable every year. And since Medigap policies provide standardized coverage regulated by the government, you don't need to worry about surprise changes to your plan each year. However, if your health care needs or income change, you may want to switch plans at some point.

If you're interested in changing Medigap plans, keep in mind:

• Unlike with Medicare Advantage plans, you are not guaranteed the right to enroll in a Medigap policy outside your initial six-month enrollment window. You can still be denied a new policy, even if you're already enrolled in a Medigap plan.

• When you switch Medigap plans, your new insurer has the right to make you wait up to six months before providing you any benefits that weren't covered by your old policy.

• Just because the government discontinues your Medigap plan, that doesn't mean you need to find a new one. Generally, your plan is still guaranteed

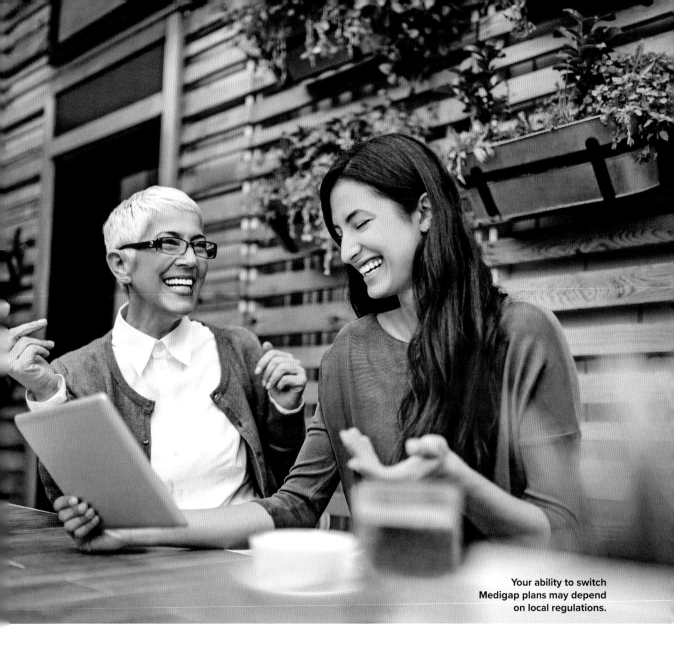

Your ability to switch Medigap plans may depend on local regulations.

renewable without any changes to your coverage, even if it isn't available to new enrollees.

• You can attempt to switch Medigap plans any time—you don't need to wait for open enrollment.

• When you switch Medigap plans, you can take advantage of a 30-day "free look" period. For the first month, you'll pay premiums for both your old and new Medigap policies. If you find the new plan isn't for you, you'll be able to cancel it and go back to your old plan.

For the most part, you'll have an easier time downgrading Medigap plans—going from a plan with more benefits to one with fewer—than the other way around. It's also worth checking your local regulations around Medigap. Some states enforce stricter protections for people trying to switch Medigap plans. ∎

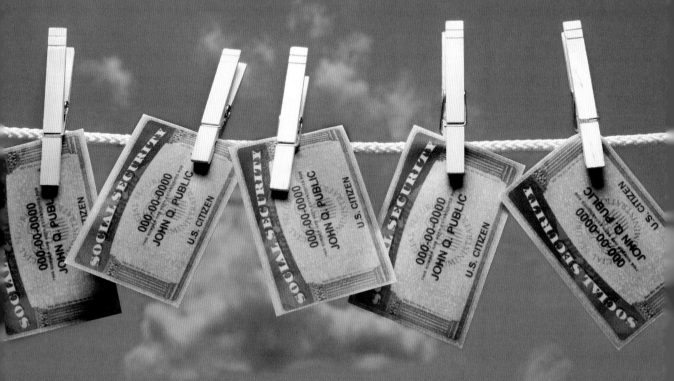

TAKE THE PAIN OUT OF MEDICARE

Social Security

What you need to know, from understanding full-retirement age to deciding when to take benefits

THE BASICS OF SOCIAL SECURITY
What it is, how you've paid in and who's eligible

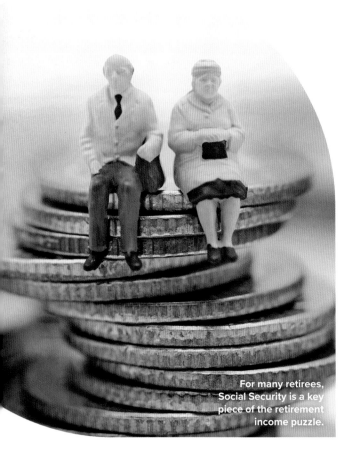

For many retirees, Social Security is a key piece of the retirement income puzzle.

Medicare wasn't America's first national program to support seniors. Old Age, Survivors, and Disability Insurance—more commonly called Social Security—started providing income for retired and disabled Americans three decades before Medicare arrived on the scene.

What It Is

Social Security is a federal benefits program that provides financial support for retirees and individuals who are unable to work due to disability. President Franklin D. Roosevelt signed Social Security into law as part of his New Deal, intended to help America recover from the economic crisis of the Great Depression; regulate business and finance; and, most urgently, provide relief to the country's poor and unemployed.

In 2020, more than 64 million Americans are receiving a Social Security benefit. Approxi-

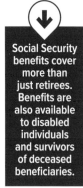

Social Security benefits cover more than just retirees. Benefits are also available to disabled individuals and survivors of deceased beneficiaries.

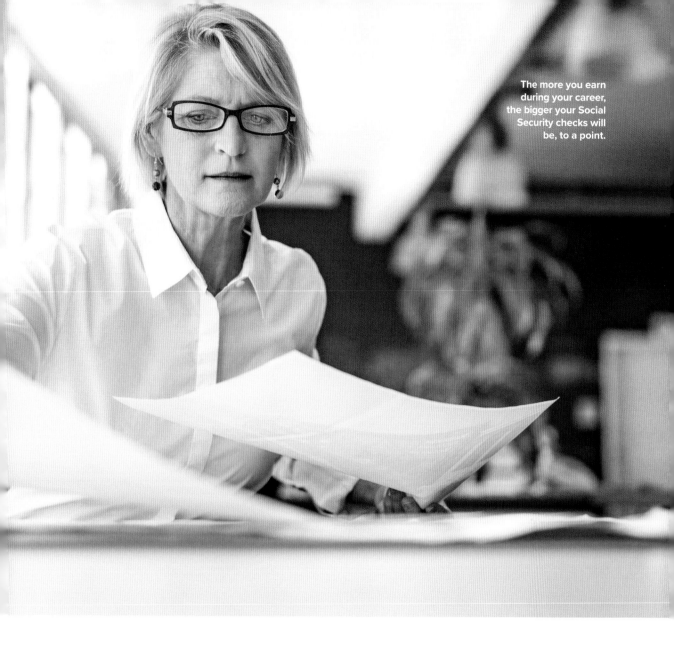

The more you earn during your career, the bigger your Social Security checks will be, to a point.

mately 48 million receive benefits because they are retired or dependents of a retiree. Another 10 million are disabled, or dependents of disabled individuals. The remaining 6 million receive benefits as survivors of deceased beneficiaries.

Who Pays What, When

When you work, you pay a tax to Social Security based on a percentage of your earnings up to a certain amount. In 2020, the first $137,700 you make is taxed at 6.2 percent if you have a conventional employer and 12.4 percent if you are self-employed. When you reach retirement age, you begin collecting monthly checks based on your lifetime earnings.

The money you put into Social Security isn't specifically saved for your individual retirement. Current workers fund payments to current beneficiaries, and leftover money goes into the Social Security trust funds.

Who Is Eligible

To qualify for Social Security, you need to meet age and work requirements. If you were born in 1929 or later, you need to accrue 40 "credits," which usually amounts to 10 years of working and paying the Social Security tax. If you stop working before you've earned enough credits, you won't be eligible. Credits don't expire, so if you come back to work after an employment gap, you will continue to build on the credits you've already accumulated. The earliest age of eligibility is 62, but to qualify for full-retirement benefits you'll need to be at least 66 or 67.

You can qualify for disability benefits at any age, as long as you've earned enough credits and you have a medical condition that meets the Social Security Administration's definition of a disability. When you reach full-retirement age, any disability benefits you receive will convert to retirement benefits of the same amount.

In certain situations, surviving spouses and children of workers can receive survivors' benefits. Surviving parents age 62 or older may also be eligible for benefits if they depended on the deceased for at least half of their expenses.

How Benefits Are Determined

While you can start taking Social Security at age 62, you may want to wait. Taking benefits later may give you more monthly retirement income.

Although Social Security began as an anti-poverty program, benefits are not based on need. Your monthly check is calculated as a sliding percentage of your lifetime earnings, adjusted for inflation: Higher lifetime earners receive a lower percentage in benefits and lower lifetime earners receive a higher percentage in benefits. Still, the more money you make over your lifetime, the larger your monthly check will be, up to the maximum benefit. In 2020, the maximum monthly Social Security benefit is $3,011, and the average benefit is $1,503.

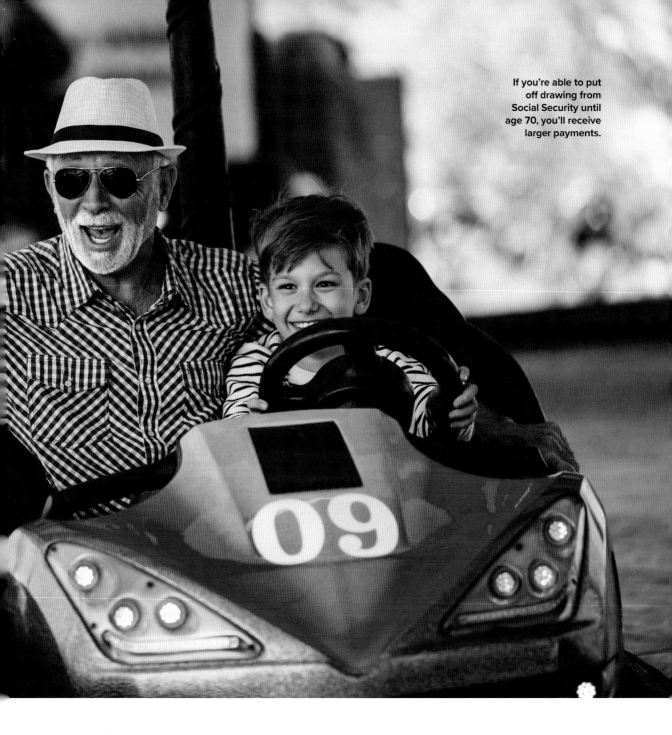

If you're able to put off drawing from Social Security until age 70, you'll receive larger payments.

Your benefit can also change depending on the age at which you retire. Depending on when you were born, you are eligible for full Social Security benefits at around the age of 66 or 67. You can choose to receive your benefits as early as age 62, but your monthly payments will be lower than if you wait until your full-retirement age. You can also decide to postpone Social Security, and your monthly benefit will then grow until you turn 70. ■

UNDERSTANDING FULL-RETIREMENT AGE
Claiming your benefits too early can be costly

When you reach full-retirement age (FRA), you become eligible to receive full Social Security benefits. For many years, the full-retirement age was 65, which is why that age is still associated with retirement in many people's minds. These days, though, most people need to wait another year or two if they want to retire with full benefits.

In 1983, Congress raised the full-retirement age for people born in 1938 or later, citing health improvements among seniors and an increasing average life expectancy. For Americans born in 1938, full-retirement age was 65 and 2 months. Each calendar year saw the age increase by two months, until it reached 66. There it paused for 12 years. Retirement age increased again, two months per calendar year, beginning with Americans born in 1955. For everyone born after 1959, full-retirement age is now 67.

Retiring Early

Even as full-retirement age has increased, the earliest age at which you can begin receiving Social Security has held steady at 62. But taking payments early comes at a cost. When FRA was 65, retiring at 62 would have triggered a permanent 20 percent reduction in monthly benefits. If you would have been eligible for a $1,000 monthly check at full-retirement age, retiring at 62 would permanently reduce that amount to $800.

As the gap between age 62 and full-retirement age has climbed, so has the penalty for retiring at 62. For someone born in 1960 or later, it amounts to a 30 percent hit. If you would be owed $1,000 a month at the full-retirement age of 67, retiring at 62 bring your checks down to $700 each—for the rest of your life. In all cases, the penalty gets milder the closer you get to full-retirement age before you start receiving benefits.

Retiring Later

If you delay your retirement, Social Security will pay you a bonus. People born in 1943 and later see an almost 0.7 percent boost to their monthly benefits for every month they wait past full-retirement age, up to the age of 70. The maximum bonus available depends on your full-retirement age. For those whose full-retirement age is 66,

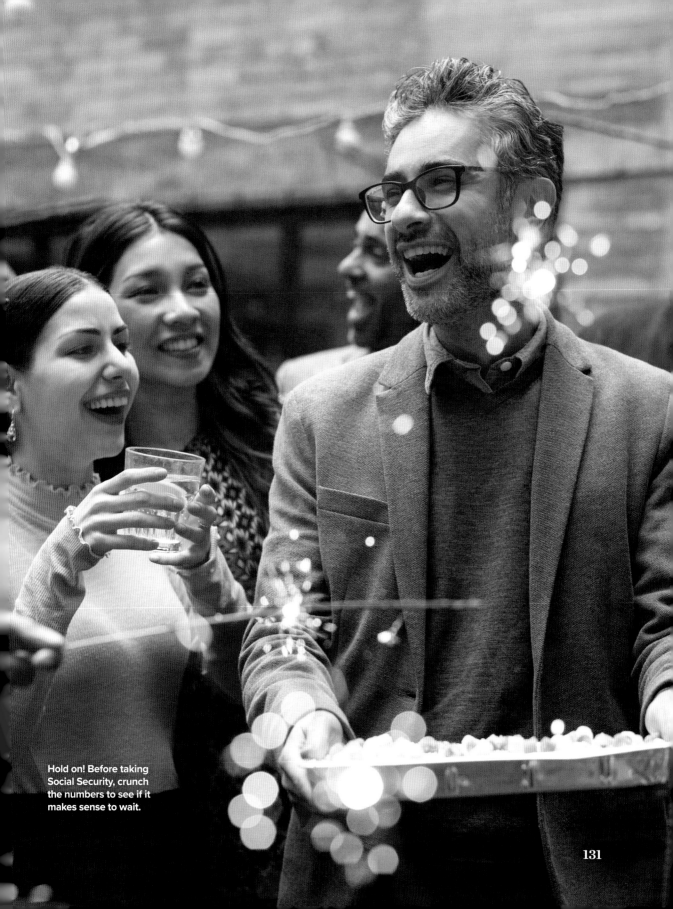

Hold on! Before taking Social Security, crunch the numbers to see if it makes sense to wait.

retiring at 70 yields a 32 percent increase in benefits. For those whose full-retirement age is 67, the same strategy will net a 24 percent bonus.

No matter when you retire, remember that you'll still need to apply for Medicare within three months of the month in which you turn 65 to avoid paying more for coverage.

When Is the Best Time to Retire?

It's impossible to generalize about the best age to begin drawing Social Security checks, but here are a few things to consider:

• **Think About Your Longevity** Because claiming your benefits early permanently reduces your benefit, doing so costs you more the longer you live. If you're healthy and your parents and grandparents lived long lives, you may, too. If you're not in good health, it may make sense to take your benefits early.

• **What Will Happen to Your Health Coverage?** Consider whether retiring early means you'll lose employer-sponsored health insurance. (Bear in mind that you don't have to stop working and claim your Social Security benefits at the exact same time.)

• **Do You Need the Money Right Now?** Getting as much as you possibly can out of Social Security is nice—but if you can't pay your bills with your current income, you may not be able to afford to wait to claim it.

• **Do You Plan to Continue Working?** Your early benefits may be reduced if you earn more income than the annual limit ($17,460 in 2019). However, there's no income limit once you reach full-retirement age.

• **In Any Case, Don't Wait Past 70** Because bonuses from delaying your retirement cease when you turn 70, waiting any longer won't gain you any additional benefits. ∎

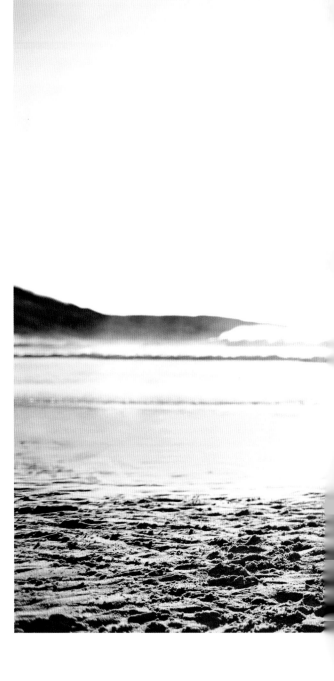

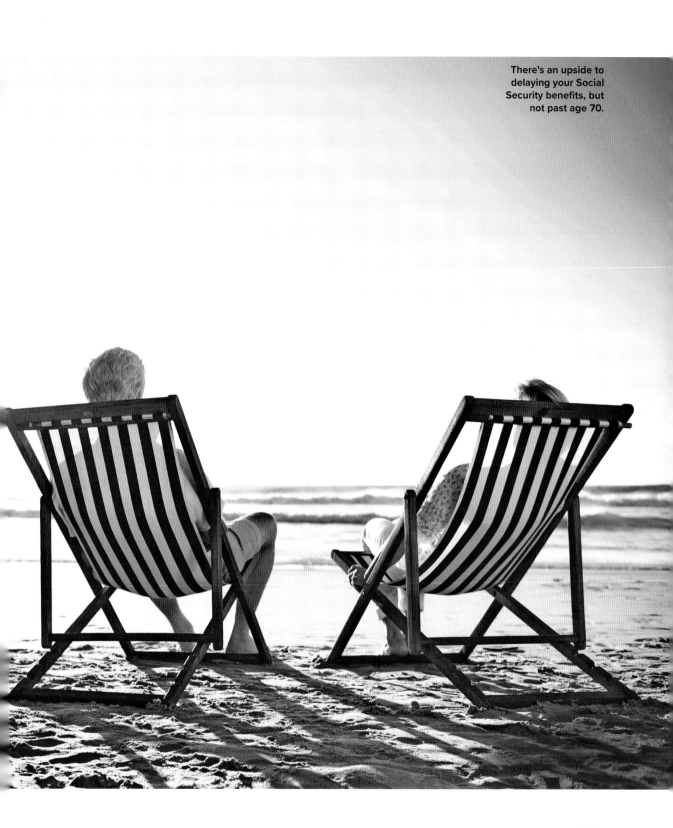

There's an upside to delaying your Social Security benefits, but not past age 70.

SOCIAL SECURITY'S PAST AND FUTURE
How it came to be, and how we keep it going

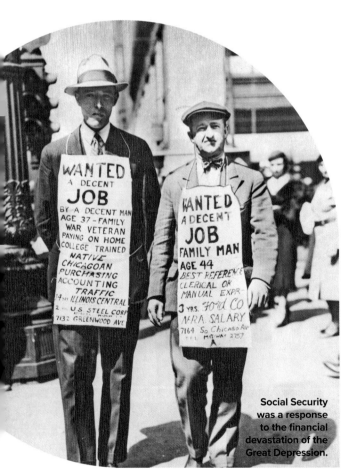

Social Security was a response to the financial devastation of the Great Depression.

In 1933, two years before President Franklin D. Roosevelt signed the Social Security Act of 1935 into law, the Great Depression hit its lowest point, with 24.9 percent of Americans unemployed. While the devastating economic decline—which inordinately affected seniors—gave the Social Security effort its intense political urgency, the financial situation for older Americans had been deteriorating for some time.

Relentless Urbanization

Americans had long been moving from farms to industrialized cities, and by 1920, 51 percent of the population was living in urban areas. People typically had no savings, so when they could no longer work, they faced troublesome prospects. Where they once might have continued working on the family farm while the younger generation took over most of the physical labor, they now were more likely to strain their children's resources in cramped apartments where almost everything they needed to exist cost money.

While wages were becoming one of the only ways to provide basic necessities, factories considered

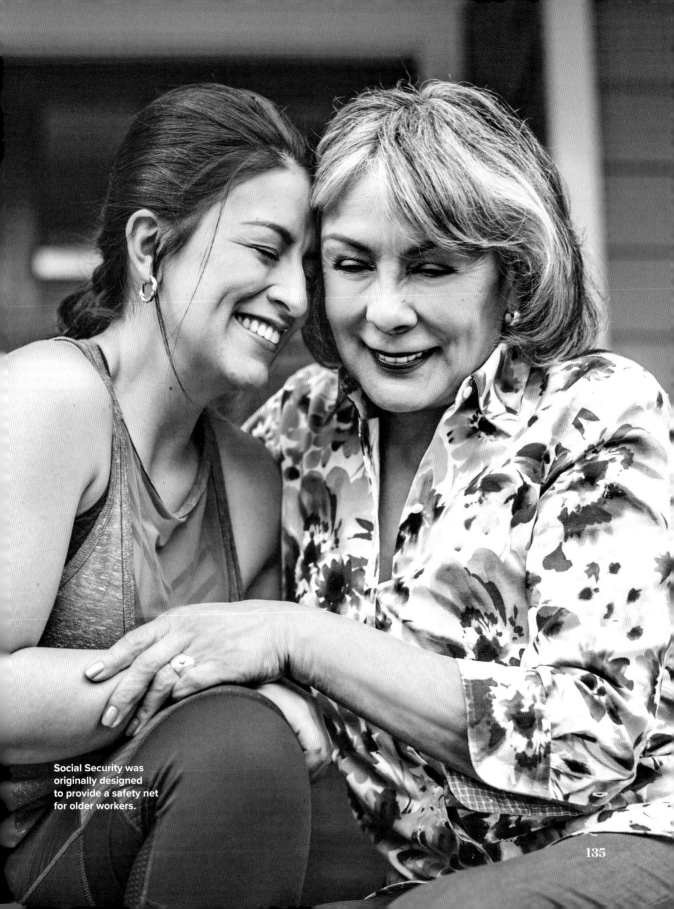

Social Security was originally designed to provide a safety net for older workers.

135

workers aged 40 or 50 too old to hire. State pension plans were unreliable and underused. As a result, many hard-working Americans "retired" to the poorhouse.

Political Obstacles

Just as Medicare was derided by opponents as "socialized medicine," Social Security, too, was cast as an attempt to "Sovietize the country." Despite the existence of social insurance programs in several industrialized democracies at the time, business interests as well as mainstream political organizations forecast bankruptcy for the United States if the Social Security tax was implemented. They also predicted that the economy would be devastated because they believed that guaranteed retirement income would eventually destroy the incentive for people to work.

Roosevelt responded with direct appeals to the American people through a series of "fireside chats" that were broadcast on the radio. In the end, a shrewd use of the bully pulpit and strong party discipline among Democratic lawmakers, who held a majority in both chambers of Congress, were enough to get the Social Security Act turned into law.

"By No Means Complete"

When it first passed, Roosevelt said Social Security "represents a cornerstone in a structure which is being built, but is by no means complete." As momentous as the law was as passed, it was still less progressive than some were calling for. Several competing bills and amendments aimed at expanding its coverage and redistributing more wealth were rejected by the House of Representatives. The program that passed was funded by a regres-

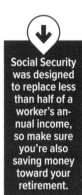

Social Security was designed to replace less than half of a worker's annual income, so make sure you're also saving money toward your retirement.

sive payroll tax, designed to replace only about 40 percent of a person's income, and benefits were not payable to the primary worker's spouse or children. Subsequent changes to the program expanded coverage or increased benefits:

- Survivors' benefits were added in 1939.
- The Disability Insurance program was established in 1956.
- Medicare was passed in 1965.
- COLAs (cost-of-living-adjustments) were introduced in 1975 as a way to match benefits to the ever-increasing cost of living without requiring special acts of Congress.

Many of the changes in the early phase of Social Security's history increased the payroll tax. Concerns about the continued financial viability of the program led to amendments in 1977 that scheduled several tax increases while simultaneously phasing in cuts to benefits. In a similar spirit, in 1983, Social Security's full-retirement age began its gradual increase from 65 to 67, which it's slated to reach by 2027.

Is It Solvent?

Arguments about the future of Social Security generally focus as much on assessments of the program's solvency as on competing ideologies about its worth. The number of beneficiaries is currently increasing faster than the number of workers. That trend suggests that Social Security's cash reserves will eventually disappear if the system doesn't change.

In its 2019 report, the board of trustees of the Social Security trust funds gave a range of possible dates by which the reserves will be depleted. Under their worst-case scenario, the combined reserves will only cover total payouts until 2030.

AARP and other advocacy groups have pushed back against the idea that Social Security is "going broke." They accept the projections but reject terms like "bankruptcy" that imply the program

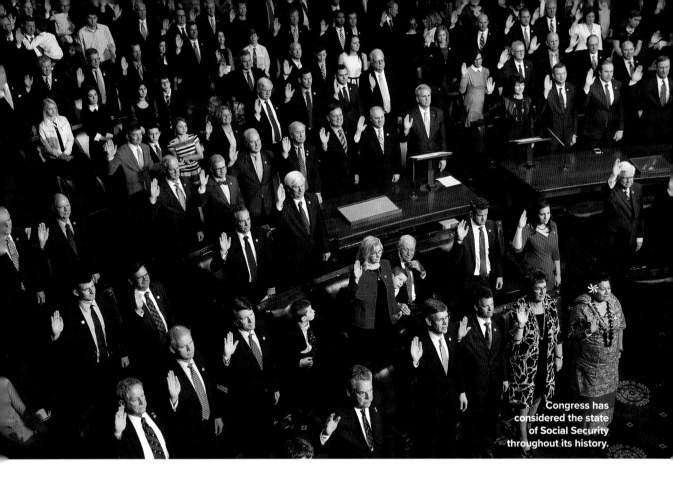

Congress has considered the state of Social Security throughout its history.

would be unable to pay any benefits. It's true that once reserves are depleted, the program will still collect revenue from the payroll tax. However, even under the trustees' worst-case scenario, income to the program would cover 70 percent of scheduled benefits after 2030.

What Will Congress Do?

The projected depletion of fund reserves provides a convenient rhetorical tool for politicians on both sides of the aisle. It can serve as proof that large social welfare programs are economically impractical, or lend urgency to a call to shore up funds to preserve benefits. In either case, it's an opportunity to renew a debate over the role of government in ensuring the prosperity of its citizens. After all, when revenues won't meet costs, increasing revenues and cutting costs can seem like equally reasonable solutions.

In 1983, the last time Social Security trust funds were in danger of dropping below the level where they could fully support scheduled benefits, Congress did a little bit of both. With four months to spare, legislators voted to phase in an older full-retirement age to keep costs down and accelerate a tax increase to boost revenue. Those changes extended the Social Security trust fund's life span by almost 50 years.

Social Security enjoys strong support among voters of both major parties. Whatever the rhetoric, it's unlikely that Congress will let the program become underfunded. But they may not be in much of a hurry to solve the problem completely just yet. ∎

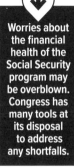

Worries about the financial health of the Social Security program may be overblown. Congress has many tools at its disposal to address any shortfalls.

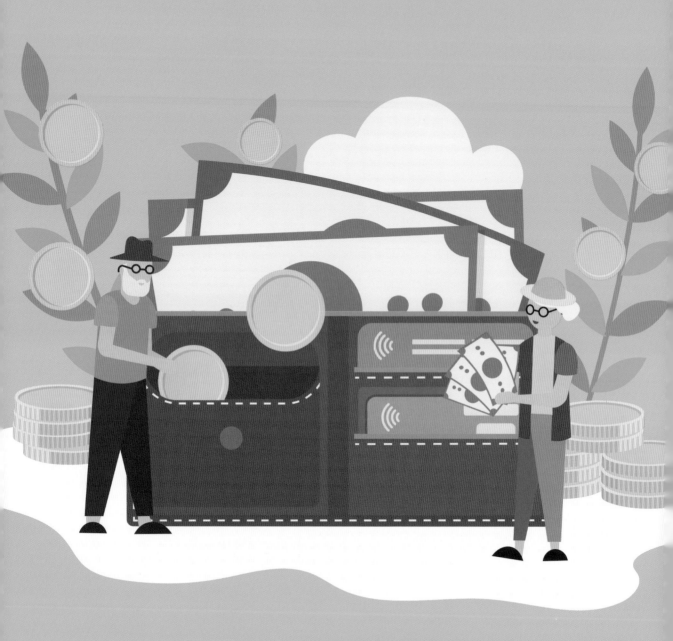

Understanding Your Benefits

What to know about how and when
to claim your Social Security benefits,
and the factors that will affect them

ENROLLING IN SOCIAL SECURITY What you need to know about how and when to apply

Now that you have an idea of what Social Security is and why it exists, you can prepare for your own enrollment. The Social Security Administration has some hard-and-fast time frames for application, but allows you quite a bit of flexibility in situations like disability or a spouse's death. It's smart to understand the timing requirements before moving on to the application process itself.

When to Apply

Two questions arise regarding the timing of your Social Security application: When *can* you apply, and when *should* you? To answer the first question, focus on your 62nd birthday—the earliest point at which most applicants are eligible for Social Security benefits. To allow for processing time, the Social Security Administration lets you apply up to three months prior to turning 62.

However, you don't have to apply at 62. For many people, it's smarter to delay filing as long as possible. That's because for every year you delay filing through age 70, your monthly benefits increase.

If you're still working when you apply for Social Security benefits, your income will factor into the Social Security Administration's benefit calculations. As a result, you'll receive reduced monthly distributions while you remain employed.

This time line doesn't apply when an applicant is disabled or is submitting an application based on a deceased spouse's retirement savings. There is no minimum age for Social Security disability coverage, and a surviving spouse can typically apply once they have turned 60.

As for the question of when you should apply: The Social Security application window opens around your 62nd birthday, but it's important not to confuse this milestone with either full-retirement age or the optimal time to claim benefits given the particulars of your financial situation.

How and Where to Apply

When applying for Social Security benefits, the first step is to gather some important information and documents. You can find the full list at ssa.gov; it includes items such as:

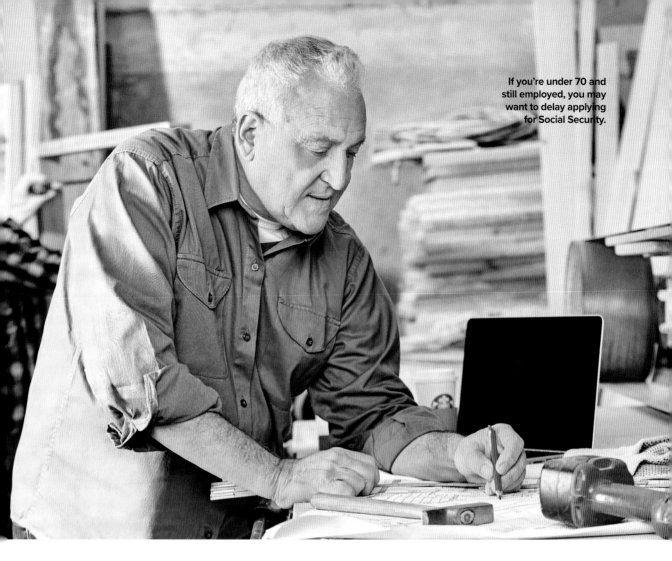

If you're under 70 and still employed, you may want to delay applying for Social Security.

- Your date and place of birth
- Details of past work experience or military service
- Information about your spouse and children
- Your bank information, so your benefits can be directly deposited

As with the age qualifications, the checklist will vary slightly for individuals applying for survivor or disability benefits.

Next, decide how you will apply. Many people will qualify for the online application process available at ssa.gov. If you have all of the necessary information on hand and are comfortable working online, this process should take about 30 minutes.

Applicants who need to (or choose to) apply in person—such as applicants with a disability—may do so over the phone (800-772-1213) or at a local Social Security Administration office. It can be helpful to have access to someone you can ask any questions you may have directly, so you can go that route if you prefer to apply with the help of an expert. An appointment is strongly recommended, but not required, at local Social Security offices.

Once your application is complete, you can check its status on the SSA website.■

SOCIAL SECURITY CLAIMING STRATEGIES
A calculated approach to applying for benefits can make a big difference over time

If you worked for 10 years or more during your life, Social Security is guaranteed income you can claim in retirement. What's not guaranteed until you actually retire, however, is how much you'll receive. Some variables are beyond your control—such as the annual cost-of-living adjustment, or lawmakers' decisions about whether to reduce or increase benefits.

However, beyond those elements, decisions that you make throughout your career and during retirement will affect your monthly check for years to come:

The primary consideration is how much money you earned over your career. That makes sense because the more you earn, the more you pay into Social Security, up to certain limits. In 2020 the maximum monthly benefit for an individual is $3,011, while the average is $1,503.

The second factor is your age at retirement—the longer you wait (up to age 70), the larger your monthly benefit will be.

Finally, if you decide to continue working during early retirement, your benefits will take a hit in the short term.

It Pays to Delay

During your career, you can always take on more work to increase your Social Security contributions, since your benefit is calculated based on your top 35 years of earned income. If you worked fewer than 35 years, unfortunately you get a big fat zero next to each of those missing years, which reduces your benefit.

But the easiest way to boost your Social Security benefit is by simply delaying retirement.

It can be very tempting to tap into your Social Security when you first become eligible to do so at the ripe young age of 62. But doing so means forgoing a larger benefit later.

If you haven't worked a total of 35 years or have one or two low-earning years, consider working longer at a higher wage to increase your benefit.

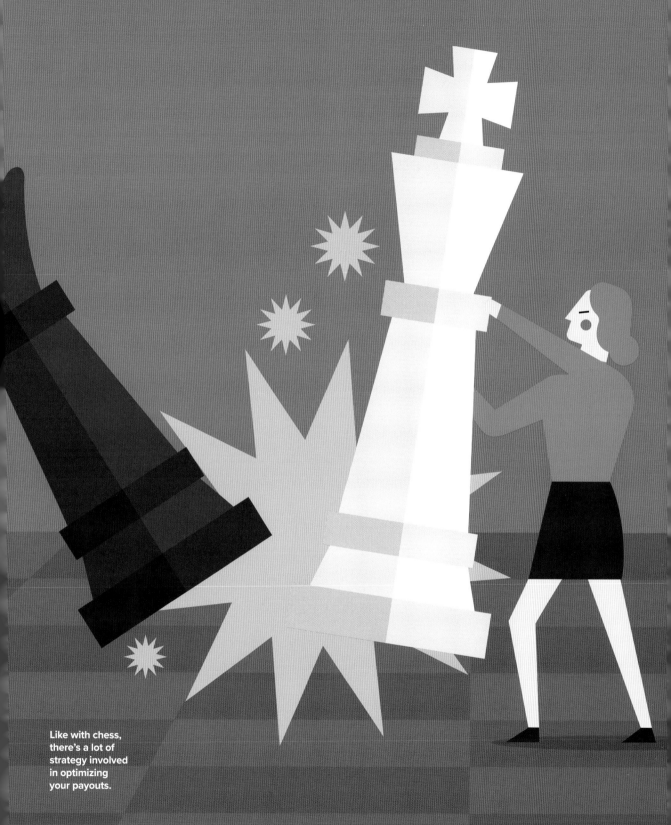

Like with chess, there's a lot of strategy involved in optimizing your payouts.

Social Security determines "full-retirement age" or FRA as somewhere between age 65 and 67, depending on the year you were born. Tapping into your benefits before FRA means a reduction in those benefits, which can be substantial—as much as 30 percent less, depending on the number of months before you reach FRA.

Conversely, you can choose to delay benefits until after your FRA, which will increase your monthly check by as much as 32 percent, depending on how long you delay. Bear in mind, though, that there is no benefit to delaying benefits past age 70.

In other words, claiming benefits early will give you a smaller check but more checks over your lifetime, whereas claiming later gives you larger but fewer checks. The choice that's right for you boils down to how long you expect to live, which most of us don't know. But if you're generally in good health and can find other ways to cover your expenses as long as possible up to age 70, it may be worth the wait.

Income from a job can affect your benefits, so you'll also need to decide whether, and how long, to keep working. A part-time job or side hustle can help you stay afloat financially in early retirement. But if you begin claiming Social Security benefits before FRA, that earned income could mean a reduction in your benefits. In this scenario—you haven't reached full-retirement age and you're earning income—Social Security will deduct $1 from your benefit payments for each $2 you earn over a set amount ($18,240 in 2020). Note that you'll get that money back after you reach FRA, in installments over 15 years.

However, if you can wait until at least FRA to begin claiming, working part-time in early retirement can potentially increase your benefits: If you don't yet have 35 years of work history, working for a few more years means you'll have more earnings on which Social Security will calculate your benefits.

Choosing the right claiming strategy can help you maximize your benefits.

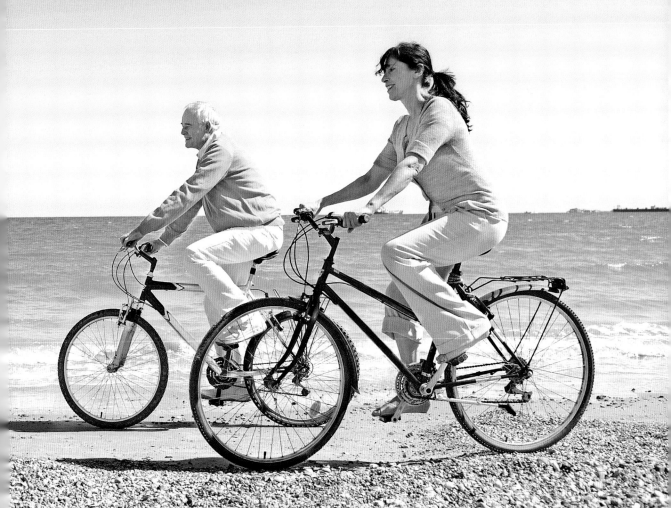

If possible, a higher-earning spouse should consider delaying benefits until age 70.

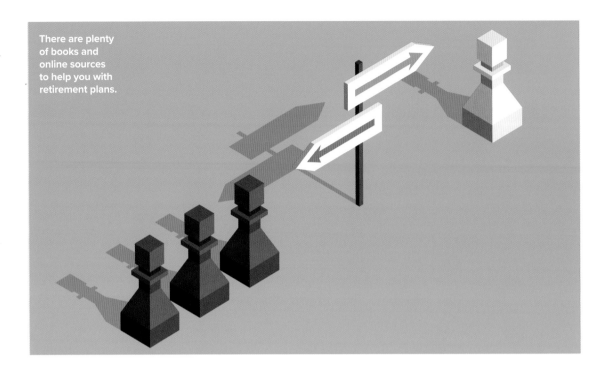

There are plenty of books and online sources to help you with retirement plans.

Claiming Strategies for Couples

For married couples, deciding when each spouse should begin claiming Social Security can be a nuanced process. Factors to consider include any age difference between the spouses, which spouse was the higher earner and whether one spouse has a limited work history.

Members of a couple who have both claimed their benefits will automatically receive either their own benefit or 50 percent of their spouse's benefit, whichever is higher. If only one spouse has filed, he or she will receive only their own benefit until the other spouse files, at which point this "deemed filing" rule applies.

> **Waiting to take your Social Security benefits can be a smart choice, so try to plan enough work or savings to give you the option to delay your claim.**

(Individuals born before Jan. 2, 1954, have the option to choose taking their spousal benefit at FRA while letting their own benefit grow until age 70—then switching. Widows and widowers of any birth date can do the same, once they reach age 60.)

Divorced couples can also claim benefits from their ex-spouses, provided:

- The marriage lasted at least 10 years
- The divorce was at least two years ago
- The spouse claiming benefits has not remarried
- The spouse whose benefits are being claimed has reached age 62

Note that the ex-spouse with the benefits doesn't need to start claiming them first—and their own benefits will never be reduced by their ex-spouse's claim.

In families in which one spouse earned significantly more than the other, the lower-earning spouse may choose to start claiming their benefits at FRA, while the higher-earning spouse puts off claiming until age 70. This strategy is

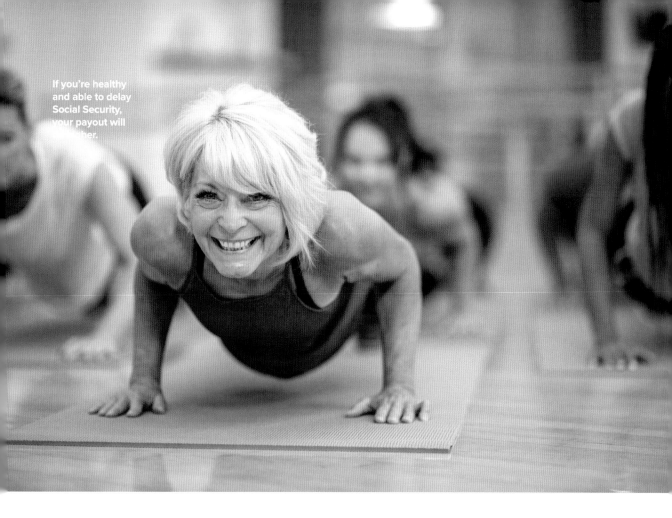

If you're healthy and able to delay Social Security, your payout will [be higher.]

especially useful if the spouses' age difference is relatively large.

For example, say a lower-earning husband with a full-retirement age of 66 gets $1,000 per month in benefits; let's also say he's six years older than his wife, whose benefits at age 70 will be $2,500. The husband could elect to receive his own benefits of $1,000 per month at age 66 until his wife starts collecting her benefits at age 70. At that point, he could switch to the higher spousal benefit of $1,250 per month (half of his wife's own benefit). Note that she will also get her full benefit of $2,500, making their total monthly benefit add up to $3,750.

If possible, a higher-earning spouse should consider delaying benefits until age 70 to take advantage of the increased benefits mentioned above. In addition to increasing the monthly Social Security benefit, this approach also increases benefits for the surviving spouse. When one member of the couple dies, the surviving spouse can elect to receive the deceased spouse's full Social Security income as a survivor benefit in lieu of their own benefits. If the higher-earning spouse dies first, this provision can create a valuable source of income for the survivor.

Taking Social Security benefits early or late depends on many factors, from your health to your spouse's benefits to your other savings. The Social Security Administration website (ssa.gov) provides many helpful calculators you can use on your own, but it's a good idea to get advice from a financial planner or tax professional. ■

HOW SOCIAL SECURITY FITS INTO YOUR RETIREMENT INCOME PLAN Strategic planning is the key to make your savings last

Social Security was never designed to be a pension plan—rather, it was meant as a form of insurance against abject poverty in old age. Fortunately, most Americans enter retirement with at least some personal resources, such as individual retirement accounts (IRAs) or a 401(k), to supplement their Social Security income. To live comfortably in retirement, you'll need to make choices about how, and when, to tap your other resources.

Your Social Security benefit is automatically adjusted annually for the cost of living. By some estimates, those adjustments over time actually exceed inflation, which gives your bank account a helpful boost. The bad news? With the average monthly Social Security payment clocking in at $1,503 in 2020, it's probably not enough to pay all your bills, which means you'll need to start tapping your savings right out of the gate. So how do you grow your nest egg and spend it? Carefully.

It may make sense to use your monthly Social Security check to pay for recurring bills like utilities, so you know you always have those covered.

Income or Growth?
With no more paychecks coming in, you need monthly income to pay bills—income that won't disappear if the stock market sinks. But you also need some growth potential to counteract inflation and ensure that you don't outlive your assets. After all, a healthy 65-year-old American could easily live another 30 years, possibly more.

The Balancing Act
Many financial planners suggest adding up your monthly bills—the stuff you can't cut back on easily, like basic living expenses and health care costs. Deduct your Social Security check from that figure, and use your savings to pay for the rest each month. Keep five years' worth of those monthly payments in a safe investment vehicle, like government bonds, at all times. You won't get much growth, but you won't lose it in a downturn.

The rest of your savings can go into riskier growth investments like stocks, since that way you'll have

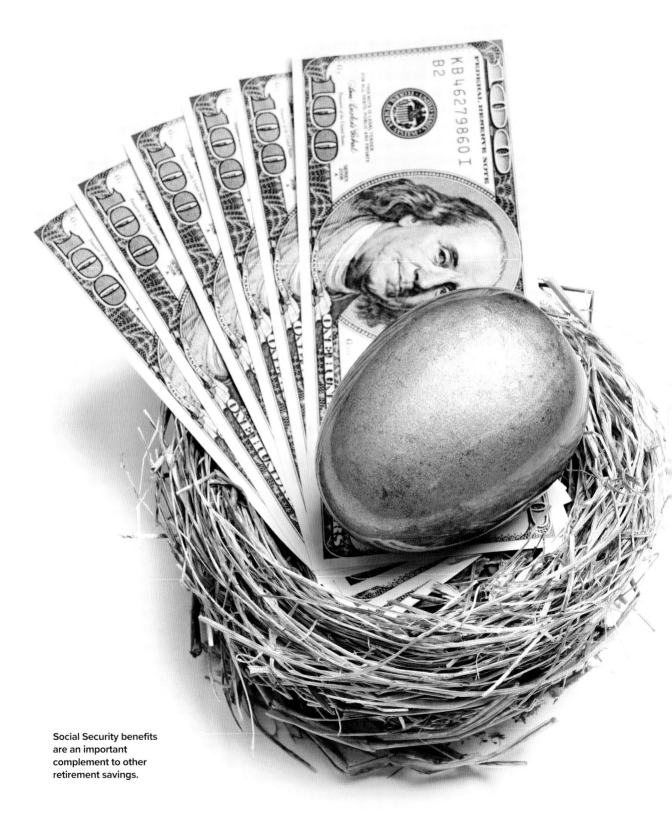

Social Security benefits
are an important
complement to other
retirement savings.

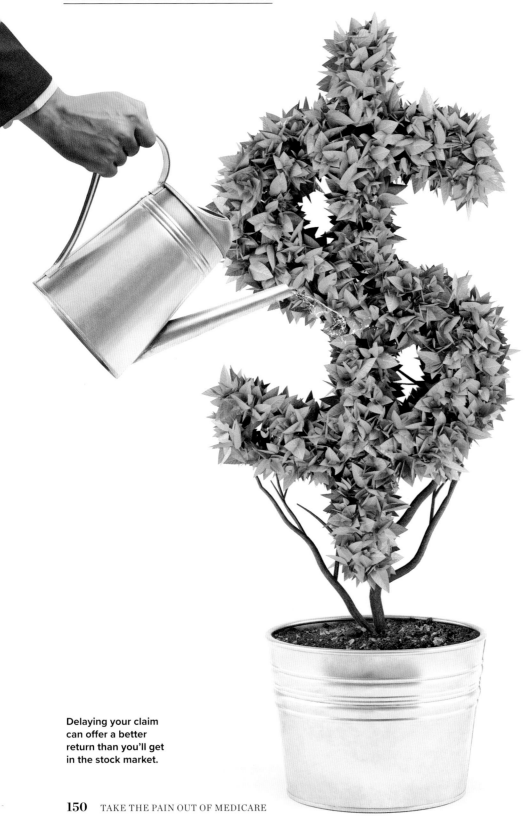

**Delaying your claim
can offer a better
return than you'll get
in the stock market.**

more time to recover any lost funds before you'll need them. As those investments grow, you'll also reduce the chances that you'll run out of money before you die.

Finding Fun Money

When you budget for your must-have monthly expenses, don't include the fun stuff like vacations, going to the movies or dining out. Use your long-term stock market portfolio to pay for those things—and only when the market has been treating you well. If the market hits some turbulence, just sit tight and wait for your savings to recover over time before you start spending money on unnecessary expenses again.

What Should I Spend First?

Conventional wisdom says to spend taxable assets (like stock and bond portfolios you've bought with after-tax income) first, and let tax-deferred assets (like traditional and Roth IRAs) grow longer. But sometimes it gets complicated, and you may pay less in taxes over the long term by withdrawing proportionally from all of your assets, every year. A financial planner or tax professional can help you make the best choice for your specific situation.

About Those Annuities...

Annuities are insurance policies that guarantee income. You pay the insurance company a lump sum out of your retirement savings, and they give you a monthly check for the rest of your life—starting either right now or later, depending on the policy.

Simple fixed annuities can be useful in a retirement plan, especially if the stock and bond markets make you nervous—but you'll sacrifice flexibility, since you usually can't take your money out of an annuity. And if you die young, your heirs won't get your money back at that point, either. Variable annuities, which claim to provide growth without risk, are typically more complicated and more expensive.

Annuities aren't insured by the FDIC, so if the insurance company goes belly-up, you could be out of luck. But many states backstop annuities up to certain amounts, typically $100,000. If the idea of an annuity appeals to you, consult a fee-only financial adviser who is not earning a commission by selling you one.

The Pension Dimension

Pensions aren't what they used to be—fewer than 25 percent of American workers have one—but for those who do, these plans can provide lifetime income. How your pension affects Social Security depends on whether your pension is private or public.

Private-sector pensions will not affect your Social Security benefit, because you paid Social Security taxes on your income. In many cases, municipal, state and federal workers such as police officers, public school teachers or court clerks are exempt from paying Social Security payroll tax since they pay into their pension fund. For them, collecting Social Security benefits would be unfair.

Laws vary by state and city, and many local governments do collect Social Security payroll tax from employees—making them eligible for both a pension and Social Security.

If an individual or a married couple has a combination of a public pension and Social Security benefits, the government uses formulas to reduce the total benefits paid out. In general, if you are entitled to both Social Security and a public pension, it's best to start taking one before the other. For example, if your pension starts at age 65, it might make sense to start claiming Social Security at age 62.

Social Security doesn't consider a pension earned income, so your pension will not reduce

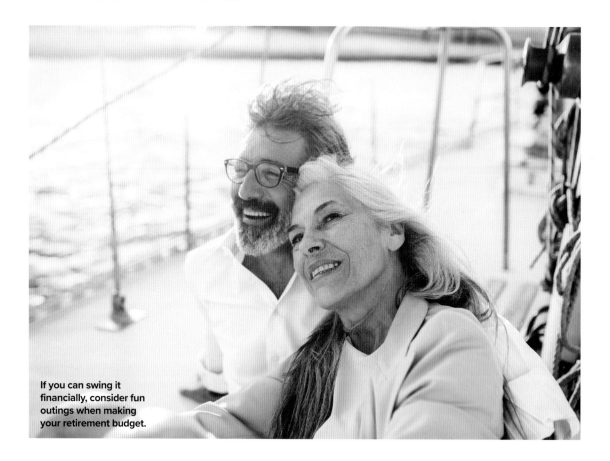

If you can swing it financially, consider fun outings when making your retirement budget.

your payments in early retirement like a salary might. But you'll likely pay income tax on your pension—and if your total income is high enough to push you into a higher tax bracket, you may wind up paying taxes on your Social Security benefits as well.

> Government workers with a pension who have paid Social Security taxes on their income may qualify for SS benefits in addition to their pensions.

Should You Invest Your Benefits?

Solid stock market returns may tempt you to claim Social Security benefits at age 62, even if you don't need the income—then simply invest the money in stocks and let it grow. But keep in mind that every year you delay claiming Social Security, your annual benefit will increase by 8 percent—guaranteed.

When Wealthy People Should Claim Early

It might be wise for wealthy people to take Social Security right away. Their monthly benefit check will be lower—but it also means less cash they'll need to withdraw from retirement funds, which could save lots on potential income or capital-gains taxes.

Since retirees spend more money in early retirement, it's a good idea to reduce taxes then when withdrawals are likely to be higher. Capital gains and IRA distributions are not considered income when Social Security calculates reductions in your benefits from age 62 to full-retirement age. ∎

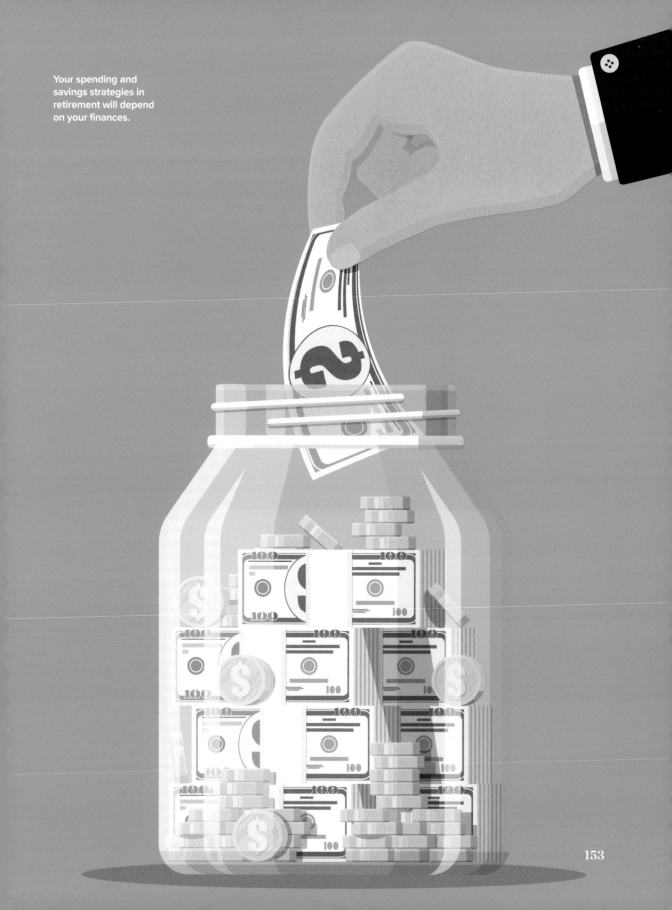

Your spending and savings strategies in retirement will depend on your finances.

HOW SOCIAL SECURITY IS TAXED
You may need to pay income tax on a portion of your benefits

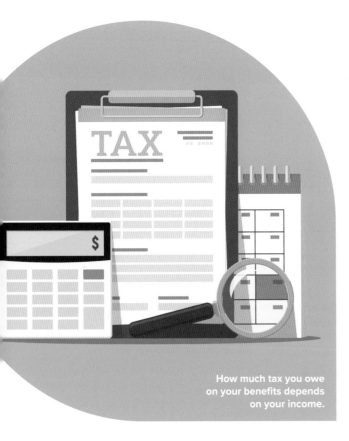

How much tax you owe on your benefits depends on your income.

Social Security retirement benefits are taxable, but how much you may owe (or whether you owe anything at all) depends on your level of income. If Social Security is your only source of income, you likely will not owe federal income taxes on your benefits. If you have taxable income in addition to Social Security, such as a salary or a pension, you can expect to pay some level of income taxes on your Social Security benefits.

How much your benefits are taxed depends on your combined income, defined by the IRS as your adjusted gross income, plus tax-exempt interest, plus half your Social Security benefits. If your combined income is below $25,000 as a single filer or $32,000 for a joint return, you won't owe taxes on your benefits. If your combined income exceeds these limits, you will need to pay some tax:

• Single filers with an income of $25,000 to $34,000 can expect to pay income taxes on up to 50 percent of their Social Security benefits for the 2020 tax year.

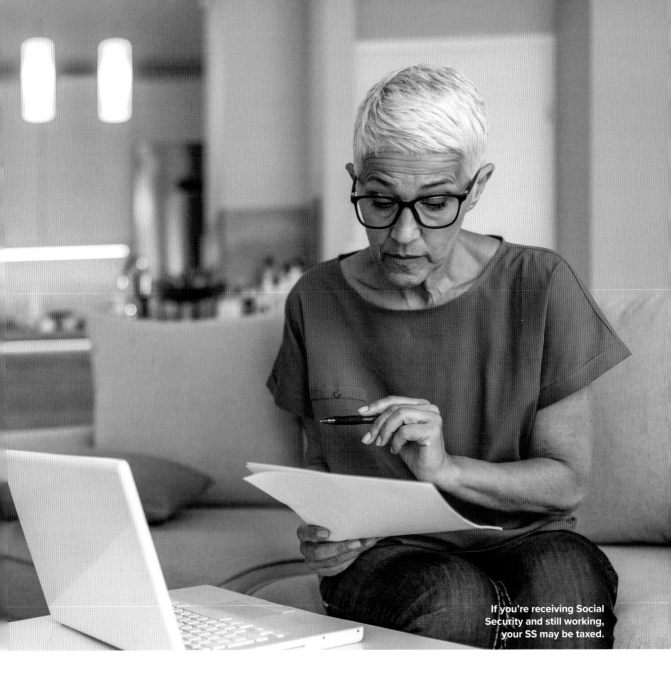

If you're receiving Social Security and still working, your SS may be taxed.

• Single filers with total income above $34,000 will pay taxes on up to 85 percent of their benefits.

• Married couples filing jointly with a combined income of $32,000 to $44,000 can expect to pay taxes on up to 50 percent of their benefits, and up to 85 percent if their combined income exceeds $44,000.

You can calculate how much tax you may owe with IRS Publication 915.

In addition to federal income taxes on Social Security benefits, you could be subject to state income taxes depending on where you live. Contact your state tax agency to learn more about how your benefits might be taxed at the state level. ∎

08	WORKING	01 | 02 | 03 | 04 | 05 | 06 | 07 | 08 | 09

RECEIVING BENEFITS WHILE STILL EMPLOYED Continuing to work after filing for Social Security can reduce your benefits

Filing for Social Security benefits doesn't necessarily mean you're ready to retire. Maybe you need to keep working to continue living comfortably, or you like staying busy and engaged. Working might make sense for your financial and personal situation—but depending on your age, your benefits may be reduced for every dollar you earn above a certain limit.

How Your Age Affects Your Benefits

You can start to collect Social Security retirement benefits at age 62, but if you file for benefits before you reach full-retirement age (FRA), the amount you receive will be permanently reduced. The size of the reduction to your benefits depends on how close you are to FRA when you start collecting payments. FRA varies by year of birth; currently, the full benefit age is 66 years and two months for people born in 1955, and gradually increases to age 67 for those born in 1960 or later. Your benefit amount could be reduced by 25 percent or more if you file for benefits at age 62.

Earned Income and Retirement Benefits

In addition to reducing your benefits if you file before reaching full-retirement age, Social Security will also subtract funds from your retirement check if you exceed a certain level of earned income for a given year. Earned income limits are adjusted annually; in 2020, this limit is $18,240. If you collect Social Security retirement benefits before you reach FRA, your benefits will be reduced by $1 for every $2 you earn over the limit. The limit on earned income disappears once you reach full-retirement age, at which point you will receive your full benefit amount regardless of any additional earnings.

Given these policies, if you plan to continue to work, it's worth thinking carefully about opting to take Social Security benefits before you reach full-retirement age. It may make sense not to, depending on what you'll earn by working. For example, say you claim early retirement benefits at age 64 and Social Security calculates your benefit to be $865 a month—about 13 percent less than your benefit would be if you waited until full-retirement age. If you decided to continue to

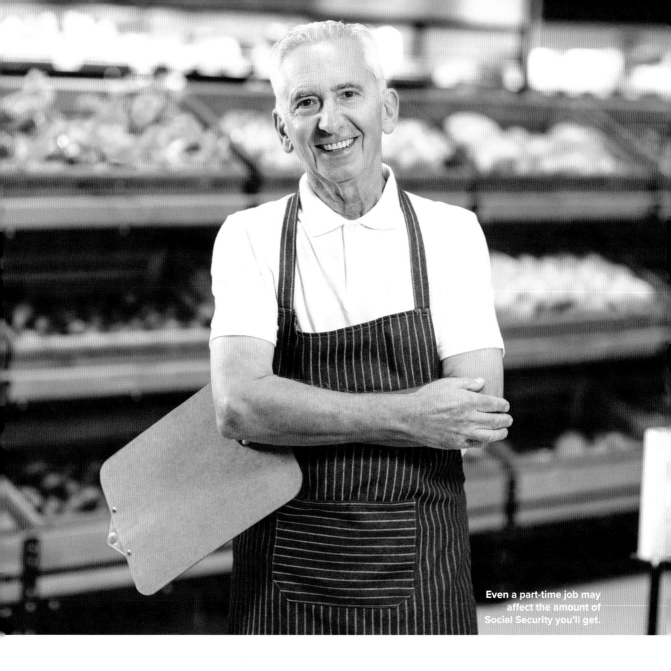

Even a part-time job may affect the amount of Social Security you'll get.

work part time at a job that brought in $23,240 for the year, you would find yourself $5,000 over the annual limit on earned income. In this case, Social Security would take half of the $5,000 you earn over the limit, or $2,500. Adding that reduction to the long-term effect of the reduced benefits you receive by claiming Social Security before you reach full-retirement age makes the situation look much less attractive.

Full-Retirement Age Adjustments

The amount you lose against your earnings is not necessarily gone forever. When you reach FRA, Social Security will recalculate your benefit amount to take into account what you lost due to the earned income limit, gradually making up for it over time. There is no limit on earned income once you reach FRA, so once you get there, you can continue to work and receive full benefits. ∎

HOW YOUR PENSION AFFECTS YOUR SOCIAL SECURITY Learn about the WEP

At certain jobs, employees don't pay Social Security taxes on wages or earn Social Security credits. These "non-covered" jobs are usually with state or local governments and come with their own government-funded pensions. (Among other non-covered jobs are certain positions with foreign companies or governments.)

Workers receiving non-covered pensions appear (from Social Security's perspective) to be long-time low-wage earners, which would set them up for higher benefits under the system's progressive payout system. Since they're already receiving other benefits, the government introduced the Windfall Elimination Provision (WEP), which may reduce their Social Security benefits. Here are the most important points:

- The WEP can't reduce your Social Security benefits by more than half the size of your pension
- The WEP can't cut your benefits to $0
- It only affects workers with non-covered pensions who also qualify for Social Security benefits

The Basic PIA Formula

To calculate your benefits at full-retirement age, also called your primary insurance amount (PIA), the Social Security Administration first calculates your average indexed monthly earnings (AIME) by taking the monthly average of your 35 highest-earning years and adjusting for wage inflation. For beneficiaries who reach the age of 62 in 2020, their PIA is equal to:

- 90 percent of the first $960 of AIME
- 32 percent of AIME between $960 and $5,785
- 15 percent of AIME between $5,785 and the maximum AIME

At this point, the Social Security Administration then applies any cost-of-living adjustments and early-benefits penalties to the PIA to determine monthly benefits.

The WEP PIA Formula

The WEP PIA alters this basic formula by reducing the factor for the first $960 from 90 percent to as low as 40 percent, depending on your "years of coverage." You earn one year of cover-

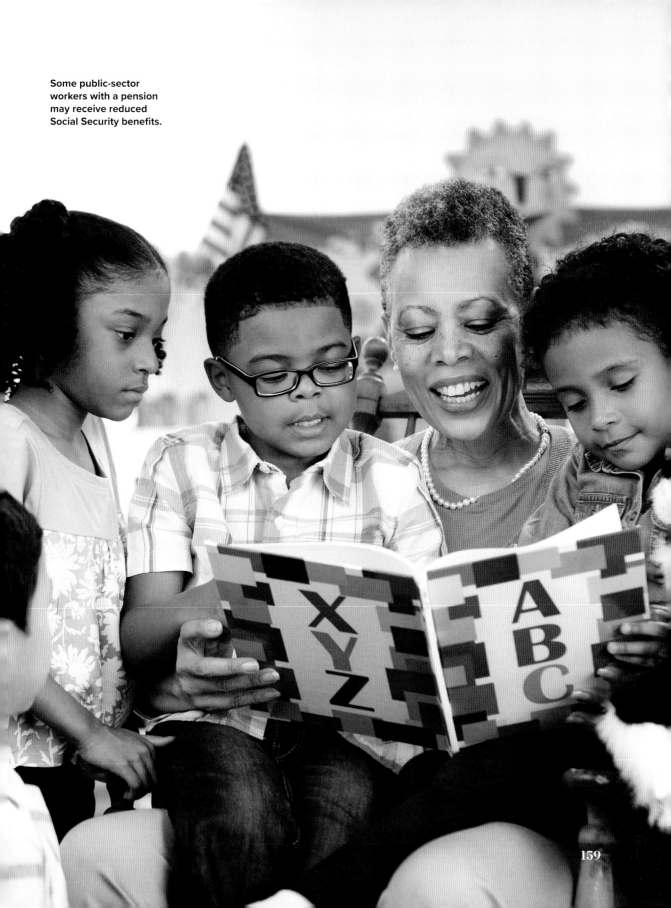

Some public-sector workers with a pension may receive reduced Social Security benefits.

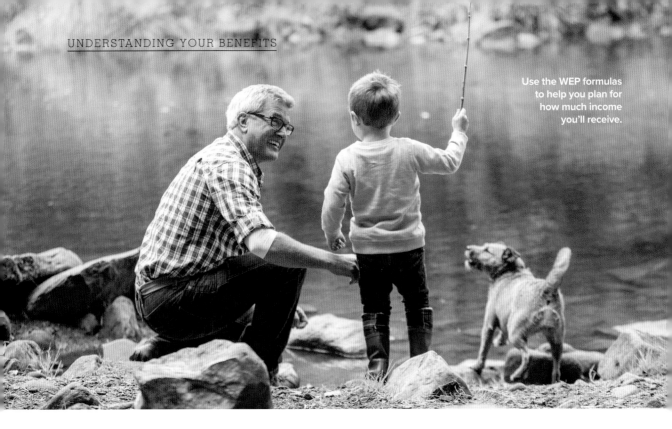

Use the WEP formulas to help you plan for how much income you'll receive.

age for every year your income from a covered job exceeds the "substantial earnings" threshold. (That threshold increases every year; see table on page 160.)

The WEP Guarantee

The WEP guarantee prevents this benefit-reduction formula from cutting your monthly Social Security benefit by more than half of your monthly non-covered pension. For example, let's say your non-covered pension pays $800 a month. Your Social Security benefit cannot be cut by more than $400 (half of $800), no matter how the formula works out.

How the WEP May Affect You

Monthly benefit calculations are so complex that the best way to learn how the WEP may affect you is to use the Online Calculator (WEP Version) at ssa.gov. There, you can enter your date of birth as well as information about your non-covered pension and the yearly earnings on which you paid

Social Security taxes. The system will then give you an estimated WEP-modified monthly benefit you can use to plan your income. ∎

EFFECT OF WEP PIA

If your years of coverage total...	...then the 90 percent factor...
30 or more	Remains 90 percent
29	Drops to 85 percent
28	Drops to 80 percent
27	Drops to 75 percent
26	Drops to 70 percent
25	Drops to 65 percent
24	Drops to 60 percent
23	Drops to 55 percent
22	Drops to 50 percent
21	Drops to 45 percent
20 or fewer	Drops to 40 percent

YOUR BENEFITS AFTER DEATH OR DIVORCE You can claim a spouse or ex-spouse's benefits in a variety of situations

Social Security is mainly a retirement benefit, but it also doubles as an important form of life insurance. If your working spouse dies, you and your children may qualify for immediate survivor benefits.

Even divorce won't disqualify you: If your ex-spouse dies, you can claim benefits on their record in many cases. If you haven't remarried, you can even claim benefits from a living ex-spouse once you reach retirement age.

Overall, the benefits after death or divorce are generous—but there's a lot of fine print involved. Here's what you need to know.

Benefits for Widows and Widowers

If your spouse dies, you can claim their Social Security benefits if you are at least age 60, or age 50 if you are disabled (generally defined as a long-term physical or mental impairment that makes it impossible to work). You can even remarry after you turn 60, with no loss of benefits. But it's important to note that you will get reduced benefits if you claim before your full-retirement age (FRA).

You can also claim the survivor's benefit at any age if you have a child younger than 16; then you'll receive 75 percent of the deceased's full benefit.

Be aware that benefit reductions last the rest of your life, so you may want to wait until you reach FRA before claiming. There is no "right" answer on when to start survivor's benefits; it will depend on your personal financial situation and other factors, such as your health and expected longevity. But in this case, it never pays to wait past your FRA.

You may also be entitled to a one-time death benefit of $255.

Kids and Parents Can Also Qualify

Children of a deceased worker also qualify for survivor's

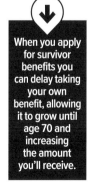

When you apply for survivor benefits you can delay taking your own benefit, allowing it to grow until age 70 and increasing the amount you'll receive.

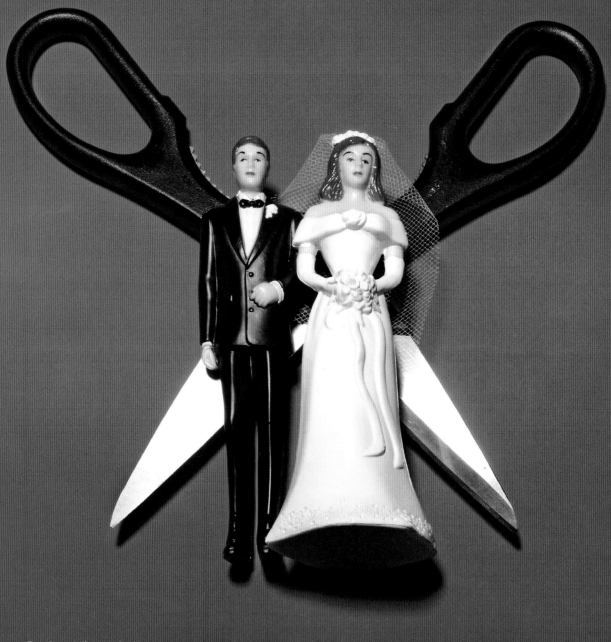

Death and divorce don't necessarily spell the end of Social Security benefits.

benefits if they are under age 18 (or 19 if still in elementary or secondary school), or disabled. Each child will receive 75 percent of the worker's full benefit.

Dependent parents who are over 62 can also claim benefits, if they have not married since the death of the worker (with some exceptions). In this case, dependency means the deceased worker was providing at least half of their support. One surviving parent gets 82.5 percent; two parents get 75 percent each. The benefit also applies to stepparents and adoptive parents, provided they became parents of the worker before he or she turned 16. In all cases, parents cannot claim both the survivor's benefit and their own Social Security benefit—but they can claim whichever of the two is bigger.

Limits on Family Claims

Before you picture a massive family windfall, note that the government limits total family benefits from one deceased worker to about 150 percent to 180 percent of the basic benefit. The actual percentage is derived using a complex formula.

When Your Ex-Spouse Dies

Ex-spouses are entitled to the same survivor benefits as current spouses, provided the marriage lasted at least 10 years and the surviving ex-spouse isn't entitled to a larger personal benefit. As with spouses, they must be at least age 60 (or 50 if disabled), or caring for a child of the deceased worker who is under 16. Note: Benefits paid to ex-spouses do not affect benefits paid to a current spouse.

Your Survivor Benefits, Explained

It's easy to see what your survivor's benefits would be. Just log on to your Social Security account at ssa.gov. (Signing up only takes a few minutes.) Follow the link to your benefits, and you'll see what your benefit would be currently, if you're over 62, as well as your benefit at FRA. You'll also see potential benefits for surviving children under 18 or surviving spouses and ex-spouses, as well as the maximum family benefit. These numbers could change every year, based on cost-of-living adjustments and your income.

After a Divorce

If your marriage lasted 10 years or more and you are currently unmarried, you can claim Social Security benefits on your living ex-spouse's work record. You will get half of your ex's benefit—which will not reduce their own benefit. You must be at least 62 years old, at which point you'll get a reduced benefit just as you would on your own Social Security record. You won't get to claim the full benefit until you reach FRA. But unlike with your own benefits, there is no advantage in delaying claiming your ex-spouse's benefits past your FRA.

If your ex-spouse has not started claiming benefits but is eligible to do so, you can still claim on their record—but only after you have been divorced two years. If you remarry, benefits end. If you become single again, benefits can resume.

No Double-Dipping

To claim benefits on an ex-spouse's record, your own retirement benefits must be less than what you would receive from your ex. For example, say you and your ex-spouse both reach FRA at 66 and your ex is entitled to $2,400 a month. You would qualify for half that benefit, or $1,200. But let's say your own personal benefit is $2,000 a month. In this case, Social Security would pay only your own benefit, and not your ex-spouse's.

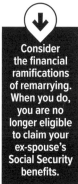

Consider the financial ramifications of remarrying. When you do, you are no longer eligible to claim your ex-spouse's Social Security benefits.

How to Claim

It's important to apply for survivor benefits right away: In many

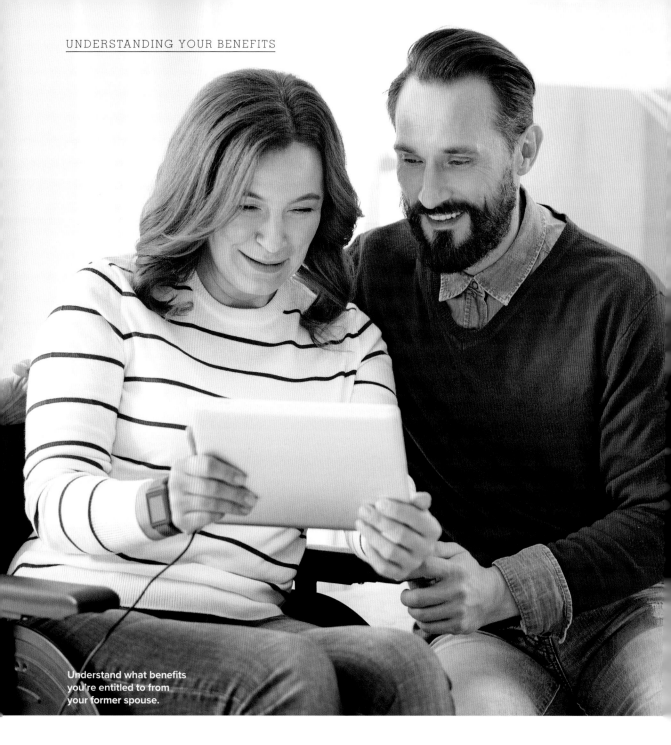

Understand what benefits you're entitled to from your former spouse.

cases the benefits begin from the date of application, not the date of the worker's death. You can't apply for such benefits online; instead, call 800-772-1213 or visit a local Social Security office.

If you are claiming benefits based on a living ex-spouse's record, you can also apply online at ssa.gov, if you are within three months of turning 62 (or older). ∎

SOCIAL SECURITY AND DEBT
When your benefit checks can be garnished—and when they can't

Transitioning from earning paychecks to receiving Social Security benefits can present a challenge when your benefits represent only a fraction of your former income. Garnishment—the legal process creditors can sometimes use to withhold money from a paycheck to force you to repay your debts—can only make it harder. Fortunately, your Social Security benefits are more shielded from garnishment than regular income is. However, the protection is not total.

Debts That Trigger Garnishment

Your Social Security checks can only be garnished to force the payment of certain types of debt. They include:

• Alimony
• Child support
• Court-ordered victim restitution
• Back taxes
• Federal student loans in default
• Some federally backed mortgages in default

In general, the kinds of debt that can result in garnishment are payments that are ordered by a court and debts that are owed to government agencies. In each case, there are limits to how much can be withheld.

After receiving a court order, the Social Security Administration can garnish up to 50 percent of your monthly benefit amount if you owe court-ordered child support or alimony and are supporting a spouse or child who is not the subject of the court order. If you don't support a spouse or child, the limit is 60 percent. And if you are behind by 12 weeks or more, an additional 5 percent can be garnished. If this formula exceeds your state's limits on how much can be withheld from income for debts, then the state limit will prevail.

The IRS can garnish no more than 15 percent of your monthly benefit to collect on a tax debt.

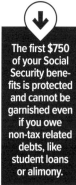

The first $750 of your Social Security benefits is protected and cannot be garnished even if you owe non-tax related debts, like student loans or alimony.

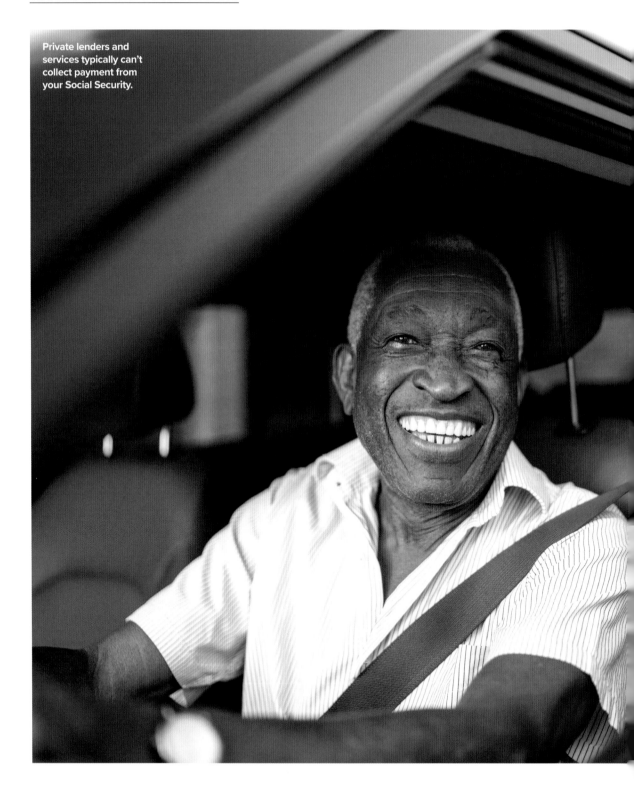

Private lenders and services typically can't collect payment from your Social Security.

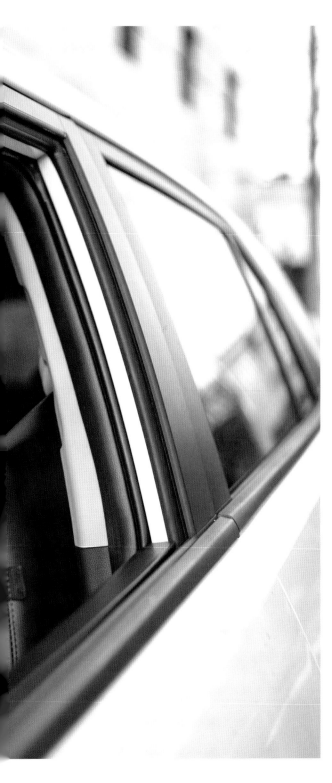

Similarly, the government is limited to taking 15 percent for defaulted federal student loans. In addition, student loan garnishments can't leave you with less than $750 in monthly benefits. Garnishment for victim restitution is limited to 25 percent.

Debts That Are Protected From Garnishment

Your Social Security income is supposed to be safe from private creditors. That is, you shouldn't be at risk of garnishment of your monthly benefit checks for things like:

- Medical debt
- Overdue car loans
- Outstanding credit card debt

That protection doesn't mean a creditor won't attempt to recover the debt some other way. If a debt collector sues you and wins, it can use a bank levy to force your bank to pay out from the money in your accounts or prepaid cards. Before complying with a levy, the bank must look through your recent account activity and protect all direct deposits of federal benefits, including Social Security, made in the past two months. With those set aside, your bank may garnish the rest.

Even then, if you believe that the money garnished is exempt, you can sue to get it back. But you will want the advice of a lawyer or legal aid office, and you may have to file quickly. While creditors are required to notify you of a bank levy, your bank is not required to do so.

Unfortunately, if your Social Security checks are garnished in error, you can't appeal directly to Social Security to dispute a garnishment. If you believe a court-ordered garnishment is in error, it will need to be challenged in court. Likewise, garnishments for debts to federal agencies, including items such as back taxes and federal student loans, must be appealed with the agencies themselves. ∎

SOCIAL SECURITY RESOURCES
Where to check your eligibility and find help

There's no one-size-fits-all approach when it comes to Social Security retirement benefits. The best time to start collecting benefits, how long to continue working, and how to reduce the impact of Social Security on your taxes all depend on your individual situation. Luckily, there are solid resources available to help answer your questions and inform your retirement decisions.

The Social Security Administration
Visit the Social Security Administration's website at ssa.gov for a general overview of the Social Security program as well as a wealth of detailed information on specific topics. The frequently asked questions at faq.ssa.gov cover dozens of areas, such as how and when to apply for retirement benefits and how continuing to work may affect your benefits.

To check your eligibility, earnings history and estimated future benefits, create a "My Social Security" account at ssa.gov/myaccount. You can also choose to apply for benefits online at ssa.gov/benefits/retirement.

You can speak with a Social Security representative over the phone by calling 800-772-1213 between 7 a.m. and 7 p.m. Monday through Friday. You can also schedule an in-person meeting with a Social Security representative by contacting your local Social Security office. To find your nearest office, visit secure.ssa.gov/ICON/main.jsp.

AARP
AARP, which was formerly known as the American Association of Retired Persons, offers advice on all things Social Security via its Social Security Resource Center at aarp.org/retirement/social-security. Visit it for detailed information on Social Security eligibility, when to apply for benefits, and tips for navigating Social Security paperwork and rules.

The resource center offers a guide to applying for retirement benefits and a benefit calculator that can show you how your retirement income changes depending on when you start claiming Social Security. The Q&A tool can also provide help by directing you to detailed information on a specific topic. ∎

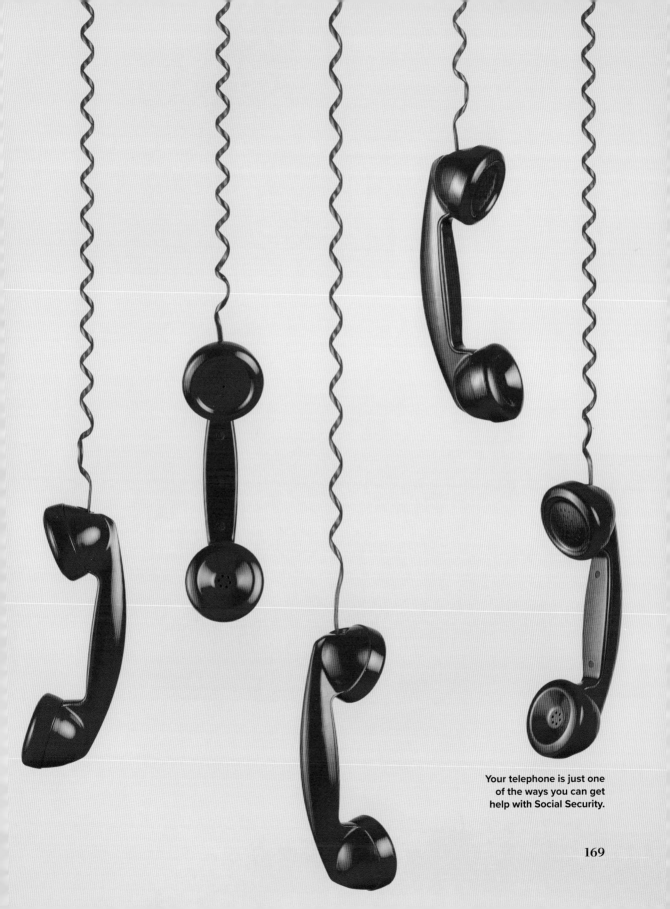

Your telephone is just one
of the ways you can get
help with Social Security.

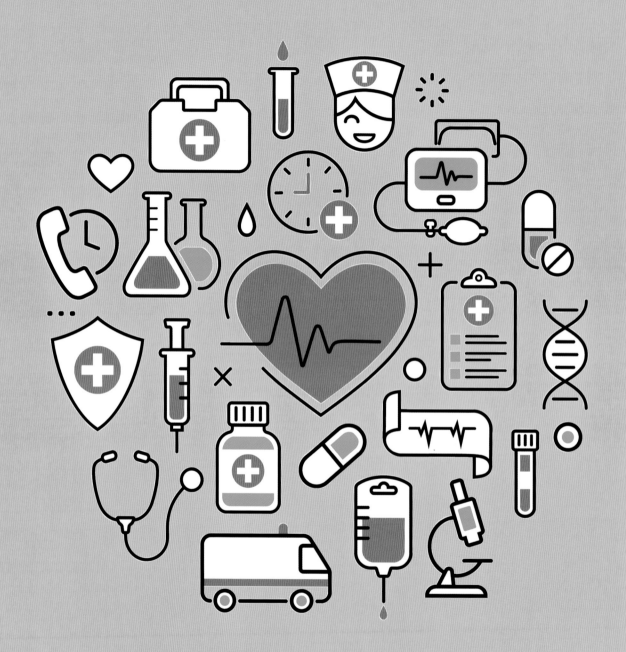

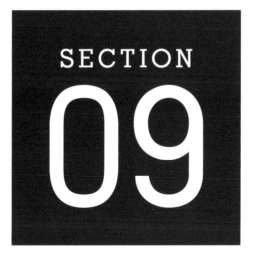

SECTION

09

Worksheets

Use these pages to plan your future and get quick facts on Medicare and Social Security

MEDICARE CHEAT SHEET
Medicare is complicated, but understanding the basics of eligibility, enrollment and what's covered can go a long way

Eligibility
• You become eligible for Medicare the day you turn 65.

• If you're already receiving Social Security before you turn 65, you'll be automatically enrolled in Medicare Parts A and B.

• Some people also qualify for Medicare based on a disability or illness.

Enrollment
Your initial enrollment period (IEP) spans from three months before the month you turn 65 to three months after the month you turn 65. Missing your IEP can bring late-enrollment penalties, higher premiums and gaps in your coverage.

Those who miss their IEP can enroll in Medicare during General Enrollment (Jan. 1 through March 31 each year). Circumstances such as losing employer-sponsored health insurance can entitle you to a special enrollment period during which you can sign up for new coverage.

You can make changes to your coverage during open enrollment (Oct. 15 through Dec. 7).

Medicare Parts A – D
Part A covers hospital services like inpatient stays, care in a skilled nursing facility, hospice care and sometimes home health care. Part A coverage is generally free.

Part B covers visits to your doctor's office and other outpatient services. For 2020, the standard Part B monthly premium is $144.60.

Part C (also called Medicare Advantage) provides coverage through private insurers. All Part C plans provide the same coverage as Parts A and B, and many include vision, hearing and dental benefits, as well as prescription drug coverage. Monthly premiums for Part C plans average an estimated $23.

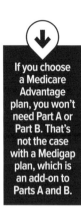

If you choose a Medicare Advantage plan, you won't need Part A or Part B. That's not the case with a Medigap plan, which is an add-on to Parts A and B.

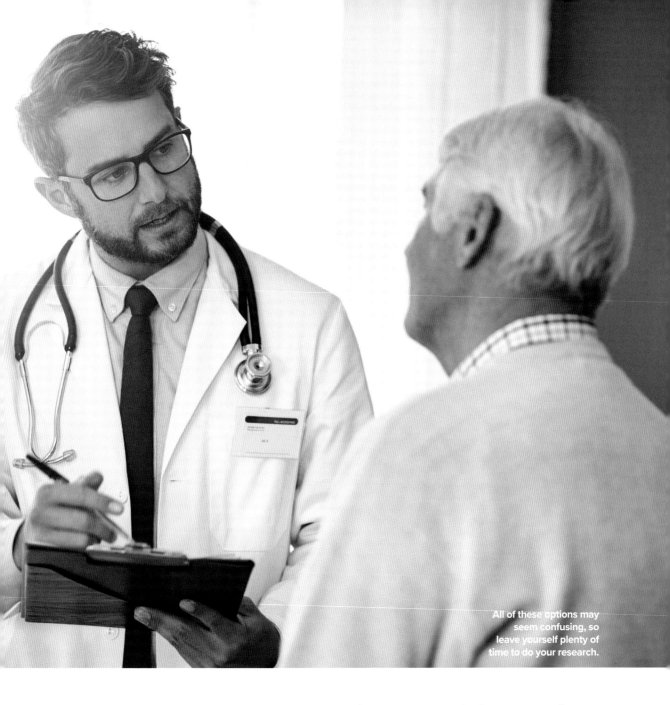

All of these options may seem confusing, so leave yourself plenty of time to do your research.

Part D pays for prescription drugs. Part D plans are sold by private insurance companies and are limited to certain geographical areas. No plan covers all drugs, so use Medicare's plan finder to locate a plan that covers your prescriptions. The base beneficiary monthly premium for Part D coverage is around $33.

Medigap Insurance Also known as supplemental insurance, it helps cover out-of-pocket costs for those with Medicare. Medigap comes in standardized plans, but is purchased through private insurers. For the first six months you're on Medicare, you can purchase any Medigap policy of your choice. Premiums vary by location and benefits. ■

MEDICARE ENROLLMENT CHECKLIST
Ready to sign up? Follow these steps to get the coverage you need

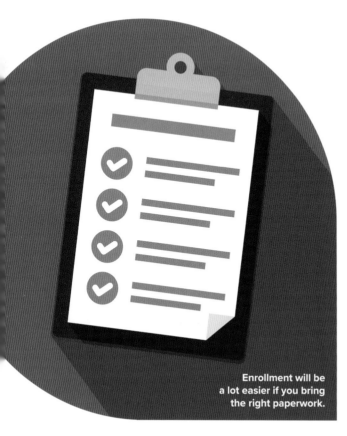

Enrollment will be a lot easier if you bring the right paperwork.

•**Know When to Enroll** By signing up before your 65th birthday, you can ensure that your coverage will kick in as soon as you're eligible. If you still have coverage through an employer (yours or your spouse's), you may want to delay enrolling until that coverage ends. If you missed your initial enrollment period, mark your calendar for the next general enrollment period.

•**Compare Original Medicare and Part C** Part C plans, also known as Medicare Advantage plans, are sold by private insurers. They can offer more extensive benefits than Original Medicare, but they limit where you can get your care. Use Medicare's Plan Finder (medicare.gov/find-a-plan) to see which MA plans are available in your area, and compare their costs to those of Original Medicare.

•**Gather Documents** To apply for Medicare, you'll need your Social Security number, original birth certificate and legal residency documents, as well as your original marriage certificate if you're married. If you've delayed signing up for Part B, you will need proof of your employer-sponsored insurance policy.

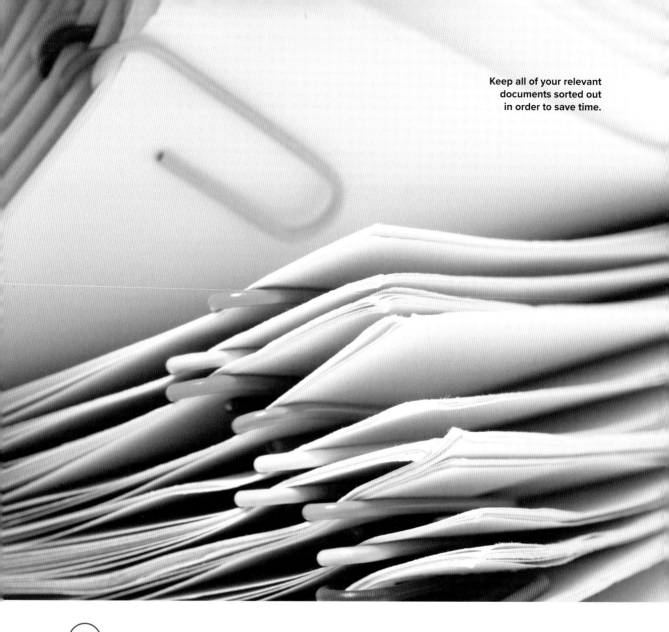

Keep all of your relevant documents sorted out in order to save time.

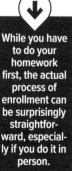

While you have to do your homework first, the actual process of enrollment can be surprisingly straightforward, especially if you do it in person.

• **Enroll** You'll be automatically enrolled in Original Medicare when you turn 65 if you've been collecting Social Security benefits for at least four months. In this case, your premium will be deducted from your benefits check. If you're not automatically enrolled, you'll need to apply online, over the phone or in person.

• **Get Supplemental Coverage** If you're opting for Original Medicare and want to add on prescription drug coverage, use Medicare's online Plan Finder to locate a Part D plan that works for you. You can also use this tool to locate a Medigap insurance policy, if you want one. If instead you've decided to go with Part C, contact the company during your IEP so you don't need to wait until open enrollment to join. Not all MA plans provide drug coverage, so if yours doesn't, make sure to sign up for a Part D plan separately. ∎

HEALTH CARE EXPENSE ESTIMATES
You can't predict what your health care needs will be, but you can prepare for monthly premiums, deductibles and copays. As you consider how to structure your Medicare coverage, compare plans by thinking about your out-of-pocket costs in various scenarios

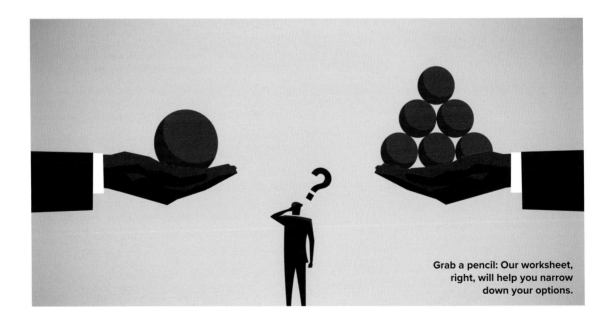

Grab a pencil: Our worksheet, right, will help you narrow down your options.

POSSIBLE COSTS	Plan No. 1	Plan No. 2	Plan No. 3
Monthly premium (including drug coverage and any supplemental insurance)			
Annual (or benefit period) deductible			
Yearly cap on out-of-pocket expenses, if any			
Coinsurance rate for inpatient care			
Coinsurance rate for outpatient care			
Out-of-pocket costs for surgery and hospital stay with a total bill of $30,000			
Out-of-pocket costs for doctor's visit for diagnostic tests totaling $3,000			

| 09 | PRESCRIPTION DRUGS | 01 | 02 | 03 | 04 | 05 | 06 | 07 |

PRESCRIPTION DRUG LIST
Keep track of which drugs you're taking and how much they cost. Save this worksheet for the next time you decide to check out your options in the Medicare Plan Finder

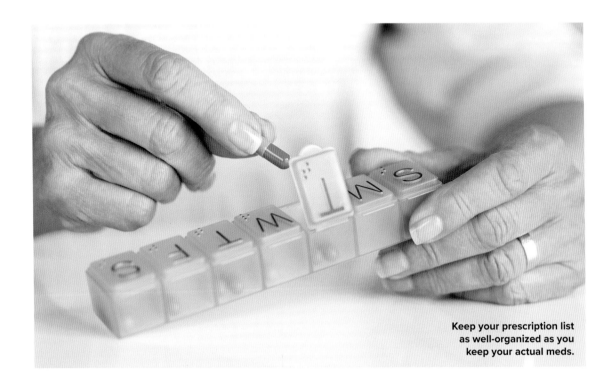

Keep your prescription list as well-organized as you keep your actual meds.

My Prescriptions	Covered By My Plan?	Monthly Cost

SUPPLEMENTING MEDICARE WITH AN HSA
Instead of cashing out of your HSA, learn how to use it to cash in

The balance in your health savings account (HSA) could become more useful after you choose a Medicare plan. Just remember to plan ahead so your balance is as large as possible—once you sign up for Medicare, you can only take money out of your HSA. You won't be able to put any more in.

Fill in the list at right and keep it with your important financial papers, and then keep your coverage information handy in your wallet, along with your Medicare ID card.

When Medicare Doesn't Cover These Costs, Your HSA Covers:
- The prevention, diagnosis, treatment and cure of any illness or defect in any function of the body
- Over-the-counter medications for which you receive a prescription
- Prescription drugs
- Transport to medical care
- Insulin medication
- Medicare or Medicare Advantage premiums
- Any deductibles
- Copayments or coinsurance payments

Your HSA Doesn't Cover:
- Over-the-counter drugs and medicines for which you don't receive a prescription
- Costs to support overall health, like vitamins, a gym membership or a vacation
- Medigap premiums ■

HSA Account Details
Provider name
Provider phone
Account login/password
Account number
Covered family members

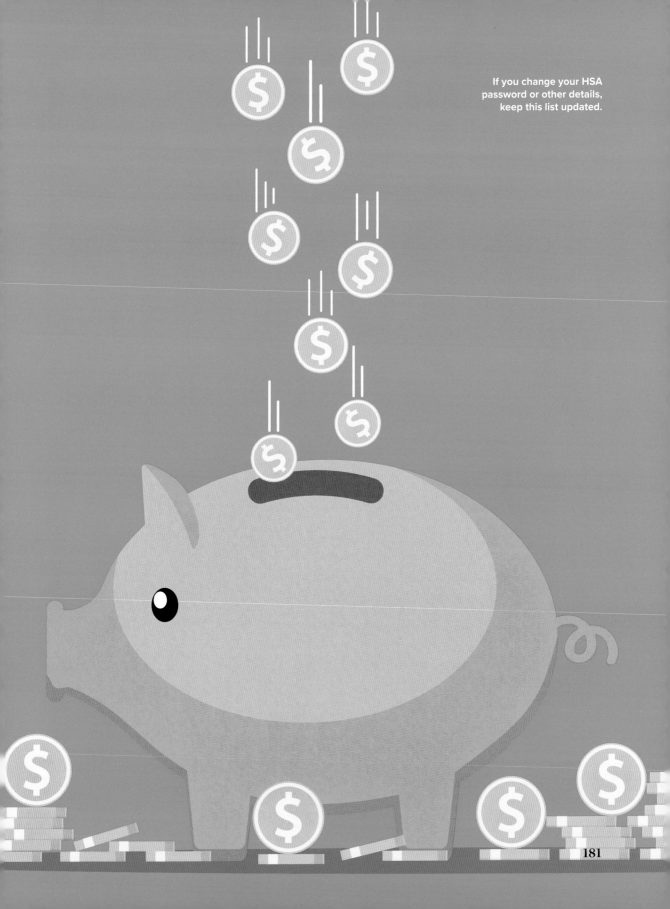

If you change your HSA password or other details, keep this list updated.

CALCULATE YOUR FULL-RETIREMENT AGE
Filing for Social Security retirement before your full-retirement age will reduce your benefits

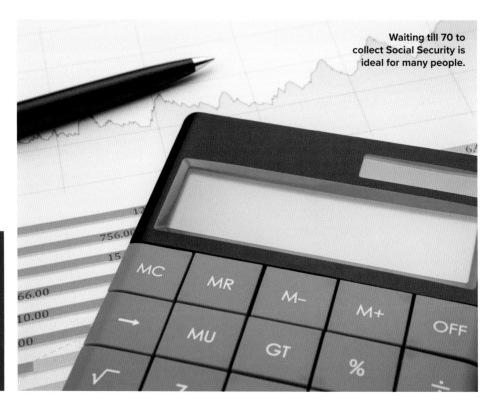

Waiting till 70 to collect Social Security is ideal for many people.

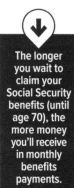

The longer you wait to claim your Social Security benefits (until age 70), the more money you'll receive in monthly benefits payments.

Knowing your full retirement age can help you decide when to file for Social Security retirement benefits.

You can file as early as age 62, but if you do, you'll receive less money each month. If you wait until your full retirement age, you'll receive your full benefits—and if you wait longer, up to the age of 70, you'll receive even more.

Use the chart to determine the full retirement age that applies based on when you were born. ∎

Year of Birth	Full Retirement Age
1937 or earlier	65
1938	65 and 2 months
1939	65 and 4 months
1940	65 and 6 months
1941	65 and 8 months
1942	65 and 10 months
1943-1954	66
1955	66 and 2 months
1956	66 and 4 months
1957	66 and 6 months
1958	66 and 8 months
1959	66 and 10 months
1960 and later	67

INCOME SOURCES IN RETIREMENT
How you'll pay for coverage once you're done working

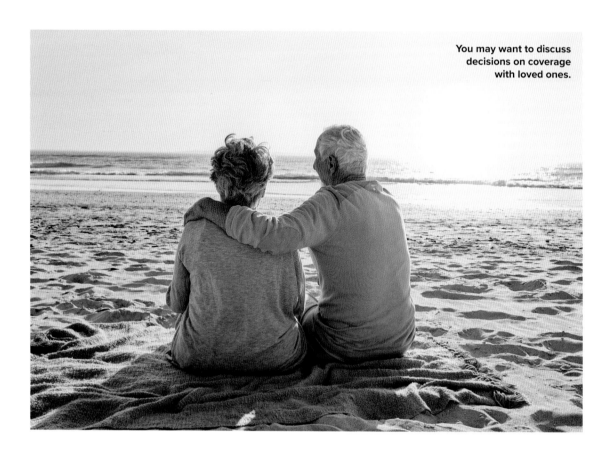

You may want to discuss decisions on coverage with loved ones.

Medicare is designed to keep health care affordable, but it's far from free. Medigap and Medicare Advantage plans with higher monthly premiums usually translate to fewer out-of-pocket expenses when you get care. However, you'll need a sound retirement plan to afford those monthly premiums. Use this chart to figure out your expected annual income, and if you choose Medicare coverage that has a high deductible or no limit on out-of-pocket expenses, make sure that your annual income can support you, even in the event of serious illness. ■

INCOME SOURCES	Monthly	Annually
Social Security benefits	$	$
Retirement plan withdrawals	$	$
Annuity payment	$	$
Pension	$	$
Savings accounts	$	$
Part-time job	$	$
Stock dividends	$	$
Other	$	$
Other	$	$
Other	$	$
Total	$	$

SPECIAL THANKS TO CONTRIBUTING WRITERS:
ERIN HEGER, BRENDAN O'BRIEN, DONNA SELLINGER, PARAM ANAND SINGH

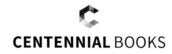

CENTENNIAL BOOKS

An Imprint of
Centennial Media, LLC
40 Worth St., 10th Floor
New York, NY 10013, U.S.A.

ISBN 978-1-951274-39-9

Distributed by
Simon & Schuster, Inc.
1230 Avenue of the Americas
New York, NY 10020, U.S.A.

For information about custom editions, special sales and premium and corporate purchases,
please contact Centennial Media at contact@centennialmedia.com.

Manufactured in China